Hairy-cell Leukaemia

Springer
London
Berlin
Heidelberg
New York
Barcelona
Budapest
Hong Kong
Milan
Paris
Santa Clara
Singapore
Tokyo

J. Burthem and J.C. Cawley

Hairy-cell Leukaemia

With 29 Figures and 7 Plates

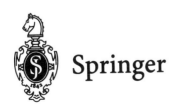

Springer

John Burthem*
John C. Cawley

Department of Haematology
The University of Liverpool, Duncan Building, Liverpool L69 3BX

*Supported by the Leukaemia Research Fund, UK

ISBN 3-540-76028-8 Springer-Verlag Berlin Heidelberg New York

British Library Cataloguing in Publication Data
Burthem, J.
    Hairy cell leukaemia
    1. Leukemia, Hairy cell
    I. Title II. Cawley, John C. (John Cozens)
    616.9′94′19
    ISBN 3 540 76028 8

Library of Congress Cataloging-in-Publication Data
Burthem, J. (John), 1961–
    Hairy cell leukaemia / J. Burthem and J.C. Cawley.
        p.   cm.
    Includes index.
    ISBN 3–540–76028–8 (hardback : alk. paper)
    1. Leukemia, Hairy cell.   I. Cawley, J.C.   II. Title.
    [DNLM: 1. Leukemia, Hairy Cell.   WH 250 B973h 1996]
RC643.B875   1996
616.99′419–dc20
DNLM/DLC
for Library of Congress   96-7343

Typeset by Wilmaset Ltd, Birkenhead, UK
Printed and bound at The Alden Press, Osney Mead, Oxford, UK
28/3830-543210 Printed on acid-free paper

Preface

In 1980, one of the authors (J.C.C.) published (jointly) a monograph on hairy-cell leukaemia (HCL) as part of Springer's Recent Results in Cancer Research series (No. 72). In the subsequent 15 years there have been enormous advances, especially in the treatment and pathophysiology of the disease. As a result, it again seems timely to review the state of knowledge of HCL. The extent of these advances has meant that a completely new book has been necessary.

The aim of the present book is to give a comprehensive review of HCL. We hope that the monograph will be useful to clinicians managing HCL, to haemato-pathologists, and to researchers interested in the later stages of B-cell development.

J. Burthem
J.C. Cawley

Contents

CHAPTER 1

Introduction and Historical Aspects

Hairy-cell leukaemia (HCL) has always attracted interest out of proportion to its frequency. Over the years, the reasons for this high level of interest have varied, but have always been underpinned by haematologists' fascination with the distinctive cytology and biology of the hairy cell (HC).

Following recognition of the disease as a distinct entity in the 1950s [33], interest initially centred on diagnosing it correctly. From the start, the diagnosis was recognised to have important therapeutic implications. Somewhat counterintuitively given the activated appearance of the HC and the frequent presence of cytopenias, the disease was recognised to behave in an indolent fashion and to be resistant to aggressive chemotherapy. Furthermore, the unusually beneficial effect of splenectomy, with its potential to produce systemic improvement, was recognised at an early stage.

Although the B-lymphocytic nature of the HC is now accepted, there was for some time considerable controversy concerning its lineage. This debate arose from the fact that the cells had a number of features thought at the time to be characteristic of monocytes, although in other respects they resembled lymphocytes. Consequently, in the 1960s and 1970s, techniques fashionable at the time (e.g. cytochemistry, ultrastructure, immunological surface markers) were used to identify the nature and lineage of HCs. Cutting a longish story short, a consensus had emerged by the end of this period that HCs represent a clonal expression of late B cells. However, it was at the same time recognised that HCs possess a number of unusual features (e.g. surface topography, tartrate-resistant acid phosphatase (TRAP) cytochemistry, unusual tissue distribution etc.) distinguishing them from other normal and malignant B-cell types.

In the first half of the 1980s, the introduction of monoclonal antibodies confirmed the clonal late-B-cell nature of HCs. Moreover, by allowing the demonstration of antigens frequently associated with cell activation, these studies resulted in the emergence of the concept that HCs are constitutively activated cells.

In the second half of the 1980s, therapy became the dominant issue, when first interferon (IFN) and then the nucleosides were shown to be especially effective in treating the disease. This in turn refocused interest on precise diagnosis, since related entities (e.g. hairy-cell variants) proved to be less responsive to treatment. Clinical experience with IFN and the nucleosides is now relatively mature, and a consensus has emerged that nucleosides are usually the treatment of choice and offer the potential of cure.

Despite this therapeutic triumph, the 'unique' sensitivity of HCL to IFN/nucleosides remains largely unexplained. The eventual solution of this problem is

likely to provide insights important to the treatment of the chronic lymphoproliferative disorders in general.

What else in the future? There is, we believe, reason to be confident that the
remaining questions relating to the disease will be answered before too long. For
example, we have recently demonstrated that HCs possess a distinctive array of
surface integrins. Furthermore, interaction of these integrins with extracellular
matrix components is probably important in the distinctive tissue distribution of the
disease. It is likely that such interactions provide signals important to the
proliferation/survival of HCs.

It is already clear that the constitutive activation of HCs is probably responsible
for a number of their characteristic features, including their unusual shape. It is
likely that this activation is related to the underlying oncogenic event responsible for
the disease. The 'HCL oncogene' may well be identified in the not too distant future.

Whatever the future holds, it is hoped that this monograph will provide clinicians,
haematologists, pathologists and researchers with a comprehensive view of this
fascinating disease.

CHAPTER 2

Clinical Aspects

2.1
Clinical features

Summary

- The disease has an incidence of around 3 cases per million per year.
- Isolated splenomegaly without peripheral lymphadenopathy is typical.
- Complications include bulky abdominal lymphadenopathy, various infections, lytic and sclerotic bone involvement, second malignancy, involvement of non-lymphoreticular tissues by hairy cells.
- These complications usually respond to IFN/nucleosides.
- The occurrence of abdominal lymphadenopathy probably represents disease transformation and is at least partly resistant to IFN/nucleosides.
- The high response rate to nucleosides has made prognostic features and staging systems of largely historical interest.

The purpose of this section is to provide a review of those aspects of HCL that primarily concern the clinician.

2.1.1
Epidemiology

HCL occurs in many different ethnic groups and has a very wide geographic distribution. The incidence of the disease has been stable over recent years and is similar in the UK and the USA (around 3 cases per million of the population, per year) [25, 338]. Typical HCL is rare in Japan, where a distinct variant of the disease is more common [208]. Otherwise, there are no geographical clues to aetiology.

Possible aetiological factors have been examined in a number of epidemiological studies (e.g. 338). Exposure to benzene, solvents and related products seems to be the most plausible of these factors. Several reports have linked the disease to such exposure [5, 110, 283, 338], but the risk has not been detected by others [258] and is, at most, modest [338]. Industrial and medical exposure to radiation has also been linked to an increased risk of contracting the disease [347] but, again, others have not found this association [338]. Other risk factors that have been cited include exposure to agricultural chemicals [110] and wood dust [338], previous infectious mononucleosis [283] and certain drugs, but all are uncertain [338]. An apparent protective effect of smoking has been noted [338], but again the significance of this observation is not clear.

Some 15 cases of familial HCL have now been described [144, 389]. Such cases are not strongly associated with any specific human leukocyte antigen (HLA), but weak HLA correlations may exist [144]. It is difficult to assess the overall significance of familial HCL, but its occurrence may lend support to the existence of aetiologically important environmental/occupational exposures. In this context, viruses have been implicated in aetiology; this subject is considered further in Section 3.6.

2.1.2
Clinical features

Age and sex distribution The overall mean age at presentation is around 50 years, with no marked difference between men and women. In contrast to chronic lymphocytic leukaemia (CLL), cases can occur in young adults. The male:female ratio is approximately 4:1.

Features at presentation Non-specific symptoms such as weakness, weight loss and dyspnoea are much the commonest reason for presentation. Symptoms attributable to infection, haemorrhage or splenomegaly cause presentation in other patients. The disease is an incidental finding in a significant minority (see Table 2.1).

Splenomegaly is by far the most constant physical finding, being present in around 85% of patients at presentation (>5 cm below costal margin in 50%). The discomfort caused by splenomegaly is usually relatively mild, and the severe pain of splenic infarction is only rarely seen. Very occasional instances of splenic rupture have been reported during the course of the disease [384]. Hepatomegaly is much less constant, being detectable in 40% of patients; hepatic enlargement is rarely marked (>5 cm hepatomegaly is seen in only 5% of cases).

In most patients there is no palpable lymphadenopathy (75%) and any lymph node enlargement is frequently limited to one node site, involving only a few small shotty glands. Even when no peripheral lymphadenopathy is present, radiological studies will reveal abnormal para-aortic glands in a minority of patients at presentation (Fig. 2.1).

Table 2.1 Symptoms at presentation

Feature	Frequency (%)
Non-specific symptoms	75
Symptoms of infection	30
Symptomatic haemorrhage	20
Incidental finding	10–20
Symptoms of splenomegaly	10

Abdominal lymphadenopathy Although uncommon at presentation, substantial abdominal lymphadenopathy may occur in up to 15% of patients during the course of their illness [34, 259, 262] and appears to be related to disease duration. The node enlargement usually involves the upper-aortic and retropancreatic regions (Fig. 2.2). This complication is now seen more often, probably as a result of patients living longer since the introduction of highly effective treatments in the mid-1980s. The hairy cells infiltrating the abdominal nodes often appear large and immature, and it

Fig. 2.1. Abdominal lymphangiogram. The lymph nodes are not markedly enlarged, but are rounder than normal and have a foamy reticulated appearance. There was no palpable lymph gland enlargement in this patient. Such nodes are readily visible on CT scanning, and lymphangiography is now of historical interest only.

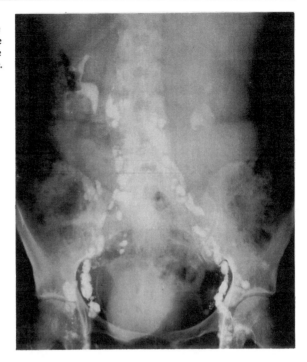

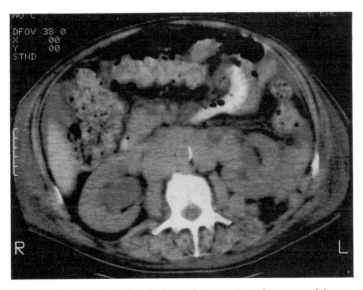

Fig. 2.2. CT scan. Massive abdominal lymphadenopathy. Extensive enlargement of the pre-vertebral nodes is illustrated.

has been suggested that this form of disease represents transformation of a type analogous to that seen in other low-grade lymphomas [262]. In accord with this concept is the fact that such patients respond poorly to treatment. They seem to be resistant to IFN and respond only incompletely to nucleosides.

Infections Before the introduction of IFN/nucleosides, infections were a major problem in HCL. Broadly speaking, infections were of two types, namely acute bacterial infections related to severe neutropenia, and opportunistic infections, perhaps associated with a more general cellular immune defect (involving monocytes/macrophages and T cells, as well as neutrophils). Since the introduction of IFN/nucleosides, infections have become much less important. However, bacterial infections may still occur early in the disease before the neutropenia has responded to therapy – granulocyte colony-stimulating factor (G-CSF) may be helpful for such patients ([132]; see also Section 6.5). Also, opportunistic infections continue to be seen occasionally [294]. A substantial list of such infections has been reported (Table 2.2), but atypical mycobacterial infection is particularly noteworthy. The mycobacterial infection may involve the lungs in a typical way, but may also present as a pyrexia of unknown origin (PUO) and be difficult to diagnose. Diagnosis may require liver or node biopsy, and empirical treatment with antituberculous drugs may be justified (reviewed in [73]). The management of PUO in HCL requires consideration of a range of possible opportunistic organisms, and also of a number of non-infective causes. Table 2.2 lists possible causes of pyrexia in HCL. The relative frequency of the listed causes is uncertain given the enormous therapeutic advances in the disease. Gram-negative organisms were the most frequent cause before IFN/ nucleosides. The opportunistic infections are now relatively more important. Only representative references for repeatedly reported infections are quoted in the table.

Table 2.2 Fever in HCL

Cause	Reference
Vasculitic syndrome	Section 2.2.2
CDA treatment	Section 6.4.2
Infection:	
Gram-negative bacterial infections	[36]
Legionella	[85]
Atypical mycobacterial infection	[252]
Listeria	[150]
Toxoplasmosis	[215]
Fungal (especially Aspergillus)	[36]

Bleeding Patients with HCL often have a qualitative platelet defect [406], as well as thrombocytopenia [73]. Nevertheless, even in the pre-IFN/nucleoside era, troublesome haemorrhage was not common. Since the introduction of effective therapy, bleeding has ceased to be a significant problem.

Autoimmune disease A number of autoimmune phenomena have been described in HCL. A systemic vasculitic syndrome is the commonest of these [105, 297, 391]; it is typically manifested as fever, arthralgia/arthritis and potential involvement of a number of organs, especially skin. The syndrome is associated with a raised erythrocyte sedimentation rate (ESR), anti-nuclear antibodies and rheumatoid factor, and immune complexes may be demonstrable [391]; its aetiology is obscure [391]. In patients with PUO, the differential diagnosis between this complication of HCL and opportunistic infection may be a key issue.

Other autoantibodies may result in autoimmune haemolytic anaemia [97], and, very occasionally, in the anticardiolipin syndrome [316] and acquired haemophilia [216]. Sweet's syndrome (neutrophilic infiltration of the skin) has been reported on a number of occasions (e.g. [86]).

The significance of these autoimmune phenomena is still not clear. They are usually, but not always, associated with active disease and disappear promptly when the disease is treated effectively. Before the introduction of IFN and the nucleosides, steroids were beneficial but they will now rarely be required.

Bone involvement Clinical bone disease is very uncommon, but radiological bone involvement does occur and may be accompanied by pain [93, 230]. Such involvement may take the form of lytic lesions [230] or diffuse sclerosis [377]. The femoral head/neck [166, 192] is a particular site of lytic lesions, while the sclerosis particularly affects the spine and pelvis [377]. Nuclear magnetic resonance (NMR) imaging is particularly useful in assessing bone involvement and its response to therapy [23]. As with the other complications of HCL, bone involvement usually responds to general treatment of the disease.

Second malignancy Instances of second tumour in HCL have been reported for many years (reviewed in [73]). However, the association seems to have become more noteworthy and is now a major cause of death in the disease. The reasons for this are not clear, but the increased survival of patients as a result of therapy may be responsible (considered further in Section 6.3.1). Overall, skin tumours of different types (basal and squamous cell, Kaposi's sarcoma and Sézary syndrome) are most frequently noted [181], but a range of other malignancies can occur, including carcinoma of the lung [181], colorectal and renal carcinoma [280] and lymphomas of both Hodgkin's and non-Hodgkin's type [1]. Finally, multiple myeloma may co-exist or develop in the disease [68]; such cases should be distinguished from the rare cases of HCL in which a paraprotein is detectable (Section 2.2.2).

Other uncommon associations A large number of other associations have been described and are probably of no particular significance given the hairy cell's propensity for tissue infiltration.

However, direct involvement of the skin [14] and of the central nervous system and meninges [228, 395] are perhaps worthy of mention since they have been repeatedly reported. Also, pleural effusions and ascites directly attributable to the disease may occur [34].

2.2
Laboratory features

Summary

- Peripheral cytopenias with variable numbers of circulating hairy cells are typical.
- The bone marrow is almost invariably infiltrated by hairy cells, but may be difficult to aspirate because of fine reticulin fibrosis.
- Diffuse hypergammaglobulinaemia is common, while paraproteinaemia is uncommon.
- Serum levels of interleukin-2 (IL-2) receptor and tumour necrosis factor (TNF) are measures of tumour burden, but add little to more conventional measures of disease activity

2.2.1
Haematology

Anaemia, leukopenia and thrombocytopenia are characteristic of HCL at presentation, and pancytopenia is present in around 70% of patients. The most variable parameter is the leukocyte count.

Anaemia Most patients are moderately anaemic and the mean haemoglobin (Hb) is similar in different large series, the overall mean being around 10 g/dl. The mean cell volume (MCV) is frequently towards the upper limit of normal and often definitely elevated. This macrocytosis is not accompanied by reduced serum B_{12} or folate levels or by marrow megaloblastosis.

A number of factors contribute to the anaemia of HCL. Measurements of red-cell mass show that it is low in only about 50% of patients, the reduced Hb level in the remainder being attributable to haemodilution resulting from an increased plasma volume [64, 232].

Splenic red-cell volume and plasma volume are increased in HCL [64, 232]. The increase in splenic red-cell volume is greater than that observed in other lymphoproliferative and myeloproliferative disorders with comparable splenomegaly [64], and this has been attributed to the great increase in the vascular space of the red pulp as a result of pseudosinus formation [66] (Section 3.2).

Radiolabelling studies have revealed that, in addition to splenic sequestration of red cells, there is some reduction in red-cell survival in the majority of patients [44, 66, 232]. There is no correlation between this moderate haemolysis and spleen size [232]. Ferrokinetic studies have shown reduced erythropoiesis in only a minority of patients [232]; however, it is perhaps worth noting that this is in apparent conflict with a number of studies showing the presence of marrow-suppressive soluble factors in the disease. The demonstration of reduced red-cell production, even if this is only slight, is a bad prognostic feature, whether or not the patient has been splenectomised [232].

Leukocytes The majority of cases of HCL are leukopenic at presentation, but a substantial number of patients have either a normal or an elevated leukocyte count.

Fig. 2.3. The high neutrophil alkaline phosphatase score of HCL. A buffy coat preparation showing the intense enzyme activity characteristically present in the neutrophils.

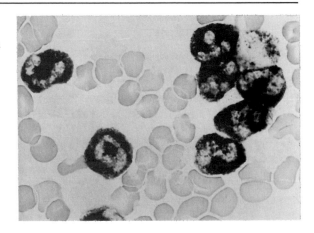

The percentage of morphological HCs varies from almost nil to l00, but in general increases with the white blood cell (WBC) count. Occasionally (~5% of cases), virtually no circulating HCs are to be found in leukopenic patients.

Most patients (>90%) have neutropenia, and this is severe (<0.5 x 10⁹/litre) in around a third. Patients with elevated total WBC counts tend to be less profoundly neutropenic; there is no correlation between neutropenia and spleen size [232]. The neutrophil alkaline phosphatase is typically increased, resulting in high leukocyte alkaline phosphatase (LAP) score [73] (Fig. 2.3). There is no corresponding deficiency of eosinophils or basophils, but profound monocytopenia is nearly always present.

Platelets Thrombocytopenia is present in >80% of patients and may be severe. Automated methods may sometimes yield spuriously high platelet counts, which should therefore be confirmed manually from time to time [341]. There appears to be no correlation between the leukocyte count and the severity of thrombocytopenia. Splenic sequestration is a factor in the thrombocytopenia of patients with gross splenomegaly [66, 232], but abnormal production of defective platelets is also observed (406).

Erythrocyte sedimentation rate The ESR is usually normal in uncomplicated HCL. Marked elevation may accompany both infections and the vasculitic syndrome that may complicate the disease.

Bone marrow aspiration The bone marrow is inaspirable or yields non-diagnostic material in 50% of cases; occasionally a dry tap at one site may be followed by successful aspiration at a second [135]. This high incidence of dry taps is usually attributed to the increase in stromal reticulin fibres characteristic of the disease.

When marrow is successfully aspirated it is usually either normocellular or hypocellular, but it may be hypercellular. The number of infiltrating HCs varies greatly and precise quantitation is difficult since they are frequently less 'hairy' than in the peripheral blood; consequently, lymphoid cells may be conspicuous. Granulocyte and monocyte precursors are profoundly reduced, while cells of the erythroid and megakaryocytic series often appear to be relatively spared.

Macrophages and plasma cells are readily found and hairy cells are not infrequently seen in close association with the former cell type (Fig. 2.4).

2.2.2
Other clinical laboratory investigations

Clinical chemistry Liver function tests are occasionally abnormal, a slightly raised alkaline phosphatase being the most usual abnormality (approximately 20% of patients). The raised alkaline phosphatase may be attributable to the periportal HC infiltration frequently present in the disease [65, 188]. The serum uric acid is usually normal, but may be raised following nucleoside treatment.

Immunoglobulins A polyclonal increase in immunoglobulins (Ig) is found in up to 30% of patients [159]; this increase most frequently involves IgG, but IgA and IgM may also be elevated [159]. Hypogammaglobulinaemia is uncommon but may also occur [159]. It is uncommon to find monoclonal Ig in the serum. Its apparent frequency depends on the techniques used for detection, but when very sensitive methods are employed low-level paraproteinaemia can be shown to occur in up to 10% of patients; monoclonal free light-chain can be detected in the urine of some 5%. The monoclonal Ig is most often IgGκ and may or may not be of the same isotypes as the surface Ig of the HC clone. It is likely that many of the low-level paraproteinaemias are not the product of the HC clone and they may represent the type of paraprotein not uncommonly found in age-matched controls [159]. However, when more paraprotein is present, this may be produced by the HCs [75], but may also indicate the presence of co-existing myeloma [68].

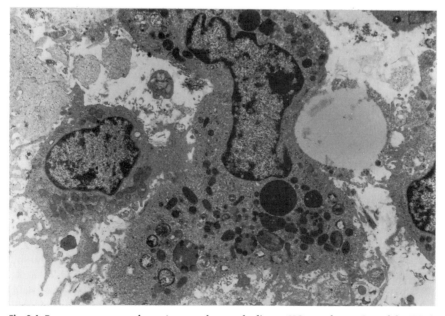

Fig. 2.4. Bone marrow macrophage. A macrophage and adjacent HCs are shown. One of the HCs is closely interdigitating with the macrophage and this is frequently observed.

The above Ig findings in HCL are in marked contrast to those in CLL, where hypogammaglobulinaemia is usual and where paraproteinaemia is considerably commoner. The reasons for these differences are not clear, but a number of factors may be relevant. For example, HCs, unlike CLL cells, have little or no propensity for plasmacytoid differentiation [e.g. 221]. Also, T cell subpopulations differ in the two diseases, CD4+ T cells being better preserved in HCL (Section 3.5.3). Finally, *in vitro* studies have shown that HCs, but not CLL lymphocytes, may be capable of secreting soluble factor(s), that, in the presence of T cells, stimulate Ig production by normal B cells (270).

Biological markers Current general interest in the clinical/biological significance of cytokines and their receptors has led to a number of such studies in HCL. Levels of IL-2 receptor and TNF have been studied most often because HCs have long been known to be unusual among B cells in expressing IL-2 receptor [217] and because TNF is a proliferative cytokine for HCs (83).

IL-2 receptor is readily shed by HCs and soluble receptor can be measured in the serum of HCL patients. Measurements of soluble receptor levels can be used as a marker of tumour burden [226, 310, 323, 344], but it is not clear that such measurements add significantly to more obvious ways of assessing disease activity.

TNF is increased in the serum of HCL patients [226, 238] and, like soluble IL-2 receptors, has been used as a marker of tumour load; IL-1β is also raised [18, 80]. In contrast, levels of M-CSF are normal [194], while those of αIFN are low [151]. It seems unlikely that measurement of cytokine levels will prove of any lasting clinical value.

2.3
Prognosis: staging systems

Before the introduction of nucleosides, the median survival in the disease was of the order of 50 months; the median survival post-nucleosides has not yet been reached. However, even before nucleosides, the range of survival was very wide and some patients were known to survive for as long as 30 years [35]; if patients lived to two years post-presentation their longer term prognosis was relatively good.

Because of this great variability, a number of staging systems have been proposed [298]. Of these, that of Jansen and Hermans [190] has been the most widely used; it related prognosis to anaemia and splenic size at presentation. Response to nucleosides is largely independent of the prognostic factors incorporated in these staging systems and, as a result, staging now seems of little relevance. The major issue now is when to start nucleoside therapy. In this regard, the guidelines proposed at the 2nd International Workshop in California (Section 6.1) seem a sensible basis for treatment; any marked cytopenia or significant complication constitutes an indication for therapy.

It is probably still worth remembering that 'spontaneous' remissions were not infrequently observed in the pre-IFN/nucleoside era [35]. Such remissions occurred mainly in patients who had undergone splenectomy and sometimes followed an episode of infection [75]. It is plausible to speculate that these remissions were induced by endogenous IFN.

CHAPTER 3

Pathology

A wide range of sites and tissues may be involved clinically or at post mortem, but the major sites of infiltration are organs of the lymphoreticular system, including the bone marrow.

3.1
Bone marrow

Summary

- Infiltration may be diffuse and complete, or partial, with islands of normal haematopoiesis.
- Cytoplasmic hairs are a less prominent feature of HCs in bone marrow; instead, well-defined nuclei separated by a clear 'halo' are characteristic.
- A variable, fine reticulin fibrosis is present.

The bone marrow is always or almost always involved in HCL, and its histology is diagnostic (Plate 1). Bone marrow biopsy material can sometimes be the means by which a diagnosis is initially made. In this regard, typical histology is the principal diagnostic feature, but confirmatory evidence may be derived from immunohistochemistry on paraffin-embedded sections (reviewed in Section 4.2), or from the TRAP activity of imprint preparations from the biopsy [218].

The diagnostic histological appearances have been described in some detail [44]. The mononuclear-cell infiltration may be partial or complete (in an almost equal number of cases). Involvement is always diffuse, although the presence of residual haemopoietic islands may in some cases give the appearance of focal HC infiltration [375]. When involvement is complete the marrow is hypercellular, fat spaces are largely obliterated and the infiltrate is seen as a monotonous sheet of relatively widely spaced mononuclear cells. Few mitoses are seen.

In marrow, the mononuclear cells do not display obvious cytoplasmic hairs. Nonetheless, they present a distinctive appearance, in which the well-defined nuclei are separated from one another by a clear zone, imparting what has been described as a halo appearance (Plate 2) [45]. This appearance has been attributed to the relatively abundant cytoplasm possessed by HCs, but also to shrinkage artefact. When involvement is complete, virtually no residual myelopoiesis is observed. When involvement is partial, the residual haemopoietic islands are composed predominantly of cells of the erythroid and megakaryocytic series. Granulopoiesis is usually profoundly depressed. Normal marrow elements from each of the three lineages may show dysplastic features [295]. Mature plasma cells and macrophages are not uncommon [73].

Electron microscopy reveals interdigitations between adjoining HCs, but the cells are frequently less closely packed than in spleen fixed in an identical manner [73, 292] (Fig. 3.1). Spaces are often present between adjoining cells. In other ways, the cells do not differ from those in the peripheral blood.

A typical and unusual feature of HCL marrow is the fine diffuse reticulin fibrosis, which is rarely seen in other chronic lymphoproliferative disorders (Fig. 3.2) [45]. The fibres associate intimately with individual HCs, and in this respect can be distinguished readily from the coarse fibrous bundles typical of myeloproliferative disorders [241]. Moreover, a significant infiltration by fibroblasts is not seen in HCL. This contrasts markedly with myelofibrosis, where a prominent infiltrate of fibroblasts produces coarse bundles composed predominantly of collagens [241]. The precise composition of the fine fibres seen in HCL bone marrow is not known; however, mature collagen is absent or minimal [269, 375], while fibronectin (FN) can be identified readily in close association with HCs [51]. We have shown that HCs have the capacity to synthesise and assemble a polymeric matrix of FN *in vitro* (Fig. 3.3), and have suggested that the malignant HCs themselves are at least partly responsible for the fibrosis that characterises the disorder [51].

Following successful treatment, regeneration of normal marrow elements may be expected. Patients achieving complete remission following chlorodeoxyadenosine (CDA) show a progressive recovery of normal haematopoiesis [100, 290]. Reticulin fibrosis appears to regress following HC elimination, but often remains present and may be found even after nucleoside analogue therapy [295].

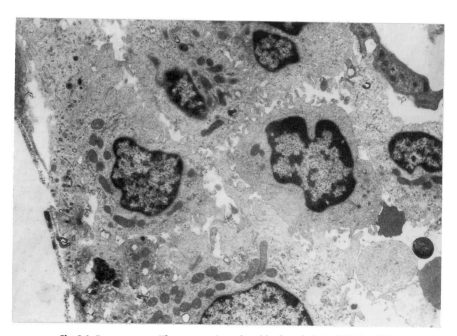

Fig. 3.1. Bone marrow. The marrow is replaced by loosely interdigitating HCs.

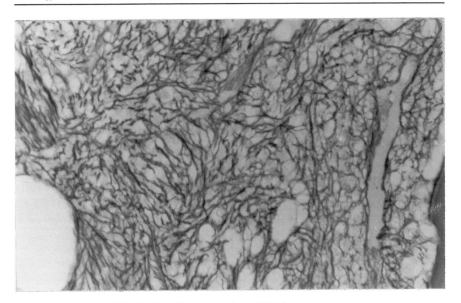

Fig. 3.2. Reticulin preparation of HCL bone marrow.

Fig. 3.3. Assembly of an FN matrix by HCs. Cells were incubated with ^{125}I-labelled FN for the indicated time. The reduced lanes (R) show that increasing amounts of labelled FN associate with HCs as time increases; the non-reduced (NR) preparations show that most of this is in the form of an 'assembled' disulphide bonded matrix.

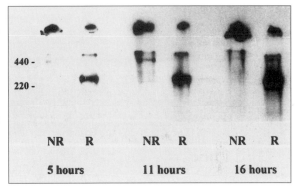

3.2
Spleen

Summary

- The spleen is always involved in HCL.
- Splenic red pulp is heavily infiltrated and normal white pulp is atrophic or lost.
- HCs pack normal sinuses, overlying and replacing endothelial cells; eventually, abnormal 'pseudosinuses' lined by HCs are formed.
- Hairs are not readily visible on light microscopic examination, but complex interdigitations can be demonstrated by electron microscopy.

The spleen is variably enlarged and generally weighs between 350 and 5000 g. The tissue is of a firm consistency, and its cut surface presents a homogeneous dark-red appearance with no evidence of circumscribed tumour; malpighian bodies are atrophic or absent. Areas of recent or healed infarction may be seen [44, 205].

Histological examination shows diffuse infiltration of the red pulp by mononuclear cells containing slightly irregular nuclei with fine stippled chromatin; nucleoli are not prominent and mitoses are not seen. The white pulp is either totally obliterated or seen as small atrophic lymphoid follicles without germinal centres, while periarteriolar lymphoid sheaths are absent. The capsule and trabeculae are not infiltrated [44, 271].

The red pulp is so heavily infiltrated with HCs that it is frequently difficult to distinguish cords and sinuses. In certain areas variably sized blood-filled spaces lined by HCs, rather than by endothelial cells, are seen in the great majority of cases (Fig. 3.4) [101, 269]. These structures, which have been termed pseudosinuses, may appear singly or in clusters presenting a haemangiomatous appearance [272]. The ring fibres that surround normal splenic sinuses are absent from pseudosinuses, but reticulin fibres of the splenic cords persist.

In addition to large numbers of HCs, the splenic cords contain readily identifiable macrophages, plasma cells and spindle-shaped cells with a compact nucleus. The macrophages contain phagocytosed cell debris. The plasma cells are not light-chain restricted and are presumed to be reactive. In addition to being scattered throughout

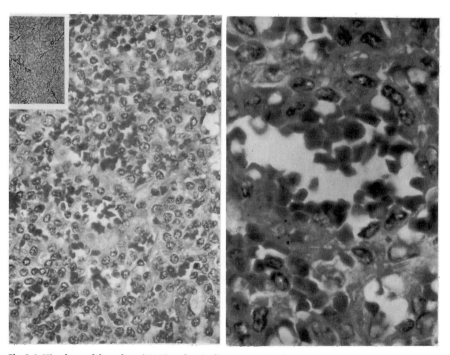

Fig. 3.4. Histology of the spleen (H&E) and reticulin preparation (inset). Vascular spaces lined mainly by HCs are evident. The inset shows that reticulin is prominent in the splenic cords but is sparse around the sinuses.

the splenic cords, plasma cells appear to be particularly numerous around blood vessels [73] (Fig. 3.5). Extramedullary haematopoiesis is infrequent [271].

Ultrastructural study has added little to basic histological observations, but has shown that the surface projections are readily evident on the infiltrating mononuclear cells. The precise appearance of these surface projections depends on the degree of packing of the HCs. When packing is loose, the hairs are relatively more prominent, but when the HCs are tightly packed the surface projections are seen as complex interdigitations, and the infiltrating cells present a syncytium-like appearance (Fig. 3.6). The cytoplasmic projections of the HCs may protrude between sinusoidal endothelial cells and through the fenestrations of the underlying basal lamina [292].

The appearances in HCL spleen are largely diagnostic, and result from the relationship between HCs and their tissue environment. HCs appear to interact strongly with the endothelial cells of spleen, attaching to them and often overlying them. As a result, splenic endothelial cells show evidence of cell injury and are eventually lost [291, 292]. This process is thought to underlie the formation of pseudosinuses by causing disruption, blockage and ultimately expansion of the existing sinus structures [272]. The resulting expansion of the intrasplenic blood compartment is probably largely responsible for the prominent red-cell pooling of the disease [306]. HCs also associate with macrophages in spleen [142]. The association of HCs with endothelial cells and macrophages may be of patho-physiological significance, since both endothelial cells and macrophages stimulate the proliferation of HCs *in vitro* [149, 36].

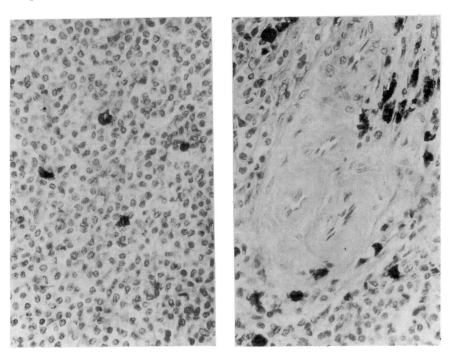

Fig. 3.5. Histology of the spleen, immunoperoxidase stain. In the left figure four strongly reactive plasma cells are seen. The HCs are unreactive on this section. In the right figure Ig positive cells surround the blood vessel. These consist of both plasma cells and macrophages.

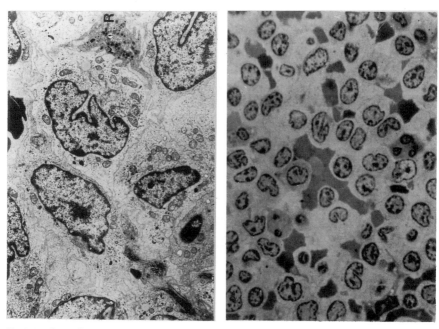

Fig. 3.6. Splenic ultrastructure. Many closely interdigitating HCs are seen. One reticuloendothelial cell is present. The semi-thin section stained with toludine blue shows diffuse infiltration with HCs which surround the vascular spaces. Some positively stained ribosome–lamellar complexes can be visualised in this preparation.

3.3
Liver

Summary

- The liver is variably infiltrated by HCs, but is not enlarged.
- Sinusoids are infiltrated by HCs, which may adhere to the sinusoidal wall in a manner resembling Kupffer cells.
- Portal tract infiltration may lead to the formation of dilated vascular spaces lined by HCs.

Exceptions occur, but the liver is nearly always variably infiltrated by HCs and its weight is frequently increased to 2500 g or more. At the time of splenectomy, the liver surface appears grossly normal, but at autopsy small nodular areas of infiltration may be seen in cut sections.

Histological examination shows a mononuclear cell infiltration of both the sinusoids and the portal tracts, but the general architecture of the liver remains intact [44, 205] (Fig. 3.7). In a minority of cases the infiltration is relatively slight, involving only the sinusoids, and may be misinterpreted as Kupffer cell hyperplasia. More frequently, sinusoidal involvement is prominent and the HCs may lie free within the lumen or in close association with the endothelium and adjacent hepatocytes. Ultrastructural studies have shown that the HCs actually attach to the

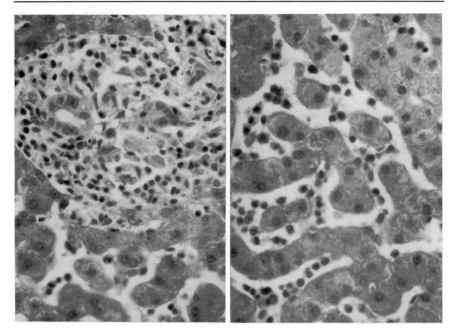

Fig. 3.7. Histology of the liver (H&E).

sinusoidal wall by means of cytoplasmic processes in a manner closely resembling Kupffer-cell attachment [90, 400].

Portal tract involvement may take the form of angiomatous lesions composed of dilated spaces lined by HCs and filled with erythrocytes [101, 272]. Although they resemble pseudosinuses, these lesions are less constant than in the spleen. The angiomatous lesions are encircled by thick ring fibres, which are continuous with those of the hepatic sinusoids. The lesions are usually confined to the portal tracts and only occasionally extend into the adjacent hepatic parenchyma. However, small similar isolated lesions with associated reticulin fibres may occasionally be observed within the hepatic sinusoids. Plasma cells are not infrequent, particularly in the portal tracts, and (as in the spleen) are reactive.

In view of this extensive involvement of the liver, the relatively minor clinical enlargement of this organ in the disease is perhaps surprising. Nor is it clear why hepatocyte structure and function are so well preserved. Nevertheless, hepatic histology, like that of the spleen and bone marrow, is diagnostic of the disease.

3.4
Lymph nodes

Summary

- Lymph nodes are usually found to be involved by HCs at post mortem, but clinical enlargement is uncommon.
- Involvement may be diffuse or focal, but residual normal tissue is usually present.

- Massive involvement of abdominal lymph nodes is seen as part of a late transformation to a more aggressive form of HCL.

Although lymph-node enlargement in HCL is rarely prominent, when node material has been examined pathologically it has been shown to be involved in most instances [44] (Fig. 3.8). Involved nodes are firm on macroscopic examination, and on sectioning they present a homogenous white appearance.

Histologically, HC involvement is variable, sometimes being seen as focal aggregations and on other occasions as an extensive diffuse infiltration of most of the node [44, 205]. However, even when massive infiltration is present, obliteration of the lymph node architecture is not total, and residual lymphocytes and lymphoid follicles are often seen [44].

Clinical infections may be associated with lymphadenopathy and, although HCs persist in the nodes, reactive changes are prominent and account for the increase in size. Plasma cells are particularly conspicuous in such nodes and display polyclonal Ig staining [142].

Considerable enlargement of abdominal lymph nodes does occur, however, in some patients, usually in post-splenectomy patients with long-standing or relapsed disease. In this group of patients, nodes are diffusely infiltrated by typical HCs, but among the typical cells are larger cells of more primitive appearance. The larger cells, which may represent blast-transformation of HCs, have an oval or kidney-shaped nucleus with prominent nucleoli. Such cells share the immunophenotypic features of HCs and may also be found in bone marrow [261, 262].

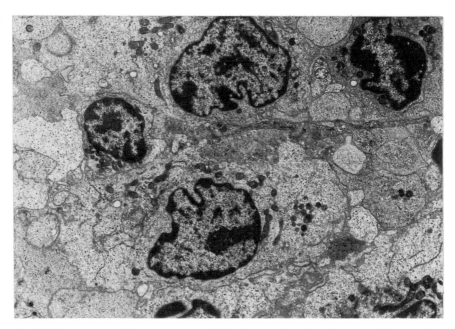

Fig. 3.8. Ultrastructure of the lymph node in HCL. There is clear HC infiltration of this node, but some of the normal architecture and at least one normal lymphocyte can be seen.

3.5
Other blood cells

Summary

- Profound monocytopenia due to defective marrow production of monocytes is characteristic of HCL; in contrast, tissue macrophages are plentiful.
- A significant T-cell population is present in HCL, both in blood and tissues; T cells may have a paracrine role in the growth of HCs.
- Abnormalities of natural killer (NK) cell, platelet and neutrophil function occur.

Qualitative as well as quantitative abnormalities of other haemic elements have been described repeatedly in HCL. Such abnormalities may have biological as well as clinical significance.

3.5.1
Monocytes

A profound monocytopenia is the most consistent and characteristic abnormality affecting normal haemic cells [37, 46], and this deficiency has been linked to the increased incidence of certain infections [252]. The almost complete absence of circulating monocytes, and of their bone marrow precursors, appears to arise principally as a result of defective production – a defect that is clearly much greater than the overall marrow suppression seen in HCL [325]. When present, monocytes have normal morphology, but may display minor functional deficiencies [325].

The mechanism that underlies the selective monocytopenia of HCL is not clear. General marrow suppression in the disease has been attributed to the secretion of suppressive factors by HCs, or to growth factor deficiencies [112, 121, 239, 355]. However, no specific suppressive factor for monocytes has been reported in HCL, and circulating levels of the principal monocyte growth factor (M-CSF) in HCL serum are normal [194].

Finally, it has been difficult to reconcile the monocytopenia of HCL with the fact that tissue macrophages are frequently abundant in the spleen, liver and bone marrow. However, in this regard, recent evidence suggests that, at least in spleen, macrophage populations are self-renewing and are not dependent on M-CSF or on replenishment by circulating monocytes [352].

3.5.2
T cells

Circulating T cells are relatively well preserved, and are present in HCL tissues. Differences have been described repeatedly between the T-cell population of HCL patients and that of normal individuals [73, 213], but the significance of these observations in the biology of HCL is unclear. HCL causes significant disruption of the normal T-cell areas of spleen and bone marrow, and secondary changes in T-cell function may therefore be expected. However, T-cell-derived cytokines are also potential paracrine growth regulators for HCs [299], and evidence has been presented that the T cells in HCL spleen are activated to secrete a range of cytokines

[213]. It seems likely, therefore, that T cells may have a role in HC growth, but the relative importance of paracrine factors compared with autocrine factors has not been determined.

3.5.3
Other haemic cells

Circulating normal B cells are significantly reduced in number, but their function seems to be well preserved [47]. A B-cell response is observed during infection, and tissue plasma cells are plentiful; furthermore, Ig deficiency is not seen in HCL and a polyclonal increase in immunoglobulins is common (Section 2.2.2).

NK cells are reduced in number and show poor recognition and killing of target cells. The deficiency is related to disease activity [342], and may be partly corrected by IL-2 [368].

Neutrophils and platelets become reduced in active HCL, and functional abnormalities of both cell types have been described [79, 406]. However, significant infection or bleeding is unusual in HCL in the absence of neutropenia or thrombocytopenia.

3.6
Viruses and HCL

Two viruses, human T-cell leukaemia virus-II (HTLV-II) and Epstein–Barr virus (EBV), have been associated with HCL; in both instances, the aetiological importance of the association is very doubtful.

HTLV-II was first isolated from an HCL patient with a prominent T-cell population [200]. Subsequently, the virus has not been demonstrable in typical B-cell disease [240]. Furthermore, populations with endemic HTLV-II infection are not at increased risk of HCL [172]. It is likely, therefore, that the virus is not important in the aetiology of HCL.

Patients with HCL have a high incidence of seropositivity for EBV antigens and the virus has been implicated in the pathogenesis of the disease [394]. However, recent serological [155] and molecular [77] studies of a substantial number of cases have failed to demonstrate the presence of EBV in HCs. It seems unlikely, therefore, that EBV is aetiologically important.

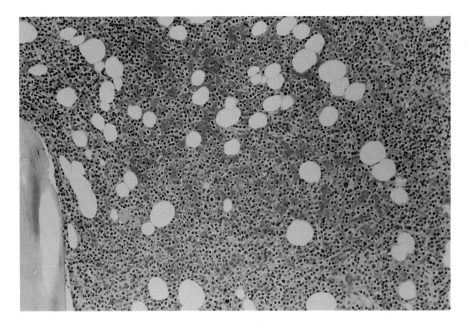

Plate 1. H&E trephine bone biopsy. The marrow is diffusely infiltrated and vascular spaces are prominent.

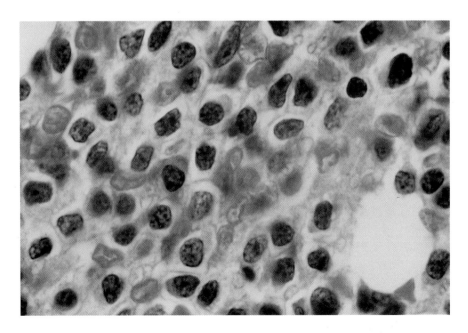

Plate 2. H&E trephine bone biopsy. The 'diagnostic' halo appearance is well shown.

I

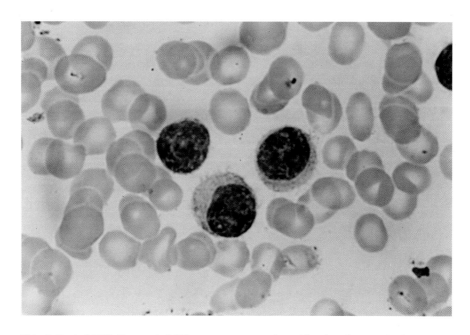

Plate 3. Typical HCL. Two typical HCs are present, together with a lymphocyte of indeterminate appearance.

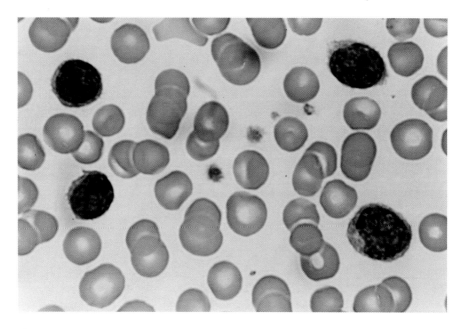

Plate 4. HCL variant.

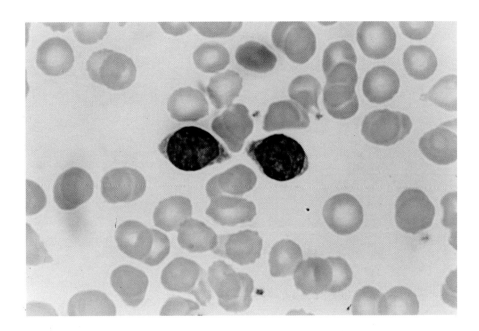

Plate 5. SLVL.

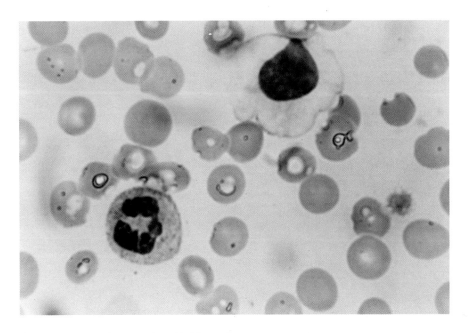

Plate 6. Japanese variant HCL (provided by Professor I. Katayama).

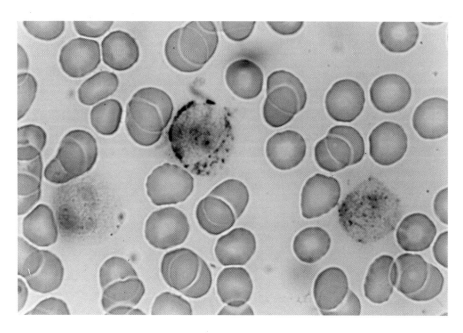

Plate 7. Tartrate-resistant acid phosphatase. Two HCs showing differing degrees of positivity are shown alongside a negative neutrophil.

CHAPTER 4

Diagnosis and Hairy-like Disorders

4.1
The diagnosis of typical HCL

Typical HCL is a homogeneous disorder. In the majority of cases a confident diagnosis can be made on the basis of typical clinical features, together with characteristic cytology/TRAP. Bone marrow aspirate/biopsy findings and immuno-cytological analysis are merely confirmatory in such cases. Clinical features (Section 2.1), cytology/TRAP (Sections 7.1 and 7.2.1) and pathology (Chapter 3) are reviewed in separate sections. In typical disease, simple immunocytological confirmation of diagnosis can be made using a panel of markers. A typical hairy cell panel is given in Table 4.1.

Diagnostic difficulties arise in two circumstances. The first is when few abnormal circulating cells are present; the second is when there are clinical or pathological atypia.

Table 4.1 A panel of Mabs useful in the confirmation of typical HCL

Marker	Reactivity
CD5	-
CD11c	+++
CD20	+++
CD22	+++
CD25	++
B-ly7*	++
HC2*	++

*These Mabs are principally used to distinguish HCL from splenic lymphoma with villous lymphocytes (SLVL) or hairy-cell leukaemia variant (HCL-V) and may be omitted in otherwise typical disease.

4.2
Diagnosis when few abnormal cells are present

In very leukopenic patients, HCs may be inconspicuous in the peripheral blood, but they are then usually identified readily in buffy-coat preparations or in the marrow. If immunophenotypic confirmation of diagnosis is required, then immunocyto-chemistry can be performed directly on smears of buffy-coat preparations. Immunocytochemistry offers the advantage that morphology and immunophenotype can be considered simultaneously. Alternatively, flow cytometry employing dual labelling may be helpful; the combinations CD19/B-ly7, CD19/CD25 and CD11c/CD19 have been advocated. It has been suggested that two-colour flow cytometry can allow identification of HCs forming as few as 1% of mononuclear cells [264, 311].

Following treatment, malignant cells may become so scanty in both blood and marrow that their identification is very difficult. This can be a problem when accurate assessment of response to treatment is required; in such circumstances paraffin-embedded bone marrow biopsies provide the most useful material. A number of Mabs have now been characterised that recognise HCs in appropriately fixed paraffin-embedded tissue; these Mabs are described in Table 4.2. It should be emphasised, however, that these Mabs all have a relatively broad specificity, and thus when used alone have a limited role in the initial diagnosis of HCL.

Table 4.2 Mabs used to demonstrate HCs in paraffin-embedded tissues

Mab	Comment
CD45/CD45RA	Anti-CD45 Mabs react with many normal and malignant cell types. However, reactivity with HCs is strong and the staining pattern is characteristic, antigen being concentrated on cell processes thereby highlighting the membrane outline and enhancing recognition in tissue sections [254]. Mabs such as 4KB5 that recognise the B-cell restricted form of CD45 offer better specificity [104], although non-reactive cases have been reported [349].
L26 (anti-CD20)	The pan-B-cell marker CD20 is strongly expressed by HCs [311]. Thus, although L26 does not specifically recognise HCs, the Mab has been used successfully to highlight HCs in paraffin-embedded tissues [104].
DBA.44	Raised against a large cell lymphoma, this antibody consistently recognises HCs in tissue sections [100]. In common with CD45 and L26, the Mab is not specific for HCL. However, unlike the pan-B-cell antibodies, DBA.44 reacts with a different spectrum of cells recognising various lymphomas, normal monocytoid B lymphocytes and some cases of monocytoid B-cell lymphoma [282, 313].
Anti-TRAP Mabs	Cytochemical tests for TRAP are unreliable in paraffin-embedded tissues [187, 349]. A recently reported anti-TRAP Mab may prove useful [187], but at present there is no general experience with its use.
Other Mabs	Anti-CD74, anti-CD75 and anti-vimentin Mabs all recognise HCs in paraffin section [282, 349, 350], but probably offer little additional advantage over the agents given above.

4.3
Diagnosis of HCL in the presence of atypical clinical or pathological features

Clinical, cytological or pathological atypia may all be seen occasionally in otherwise typical HCL. Therapeutic and prognostic reasons mean that it is important to discriminate accurately between atypical presentations of HCL and related disorders. Again, it should be emphasised that accurate diagnosis depends on the overall consideration of clinical, pathological and immunological features. In the latter regard, immunocytology provides useful and objective diagnostic information. It

Table 4.3 Immunological surface markers useful in the evaluation of HCL

Marker	Level	Comment
		Important non-hairy-cell markers
CD3	-	CD3 is not expressed by typical HCL, although rare cases simultaneously expressing B- and T -cell characteristics have been described [16, 91].
CD5	-	HCL does not normally express CD5, although this antigen is expressed in a proportion of cases of HCL-V [257] and in very rare cases of typical HCL [165]. CD5 reactivity is generally useful in distinguishing between typical HCL and CLL.
		General B-lymphocyte markers
CD19/20	+/+++	HCs react with both these pan B-cell markers. CD20 is significantly more strongly expressed [311].
CD38	±	Although not generally expressed, this plasma cell marker may be expressed on a proportion (~10%) of cases of typical HCL [257].
FMC7	+++	HCs consistently react with this differentiation antigen, but the antigen is also expressed in related disorders, and quantitatively similar levels are detected on HCs and PLL cells [26].
κ/λ light chains	+++	Strong, light-chain-restricted sIg is characteristic of HCL, but also occurs in related disorders. κ/λ ratios are approximately equal [48, 191, 211].
		'Specific' hairy-cell markers
CD11c	++++	Strong CD11c expression is characteristic of typical HCL [379], but the antigen is also strongly expressed by normal monocytes and NK cells. More importantly, the antigen is expressed at low to moderate levels in 90% of PLL and in up to 30% of CLL patients [214]. CD11c can be a useful marker of HCL, but must be strongly expressed, preferably in conjunction with other specific markers. The antigen is of less use in distinguishing between HCL and closely related disorders (Table 4.6).
CD22	++++	Intense surface expression of CD22 is typical of HCL. However, CD22 Mabs also recognise a range of other normal and malignant B cells; strong reactivity may be seen in cases of PLL or follicular and mantle lymphomas [214]. Nonetheless, strong quantitative expression of CD22, particularly in combination with more specific markers, is very useful in the diagnosis of HCL [264, 311].
CD25	++	CD25 is less strongly expressed than CD22 or CD11c, but all, or nearly all, cases of typical HCL express at least moderate levels of the antigen [257, 311]. CD25 is also expressed by activated B and T cells and by NK cells. Up to 25% of CLL patients express the antigen at low intensity [214]. CD25 expression is useful in differentiating HCL from HCL-V (Table 4.6).
B-ly7	++	B-ly7 recognises the integrin complex αHβ7 (CD103, HML-l antigen). Expression of the integrin is restricted to certain mucosal T lymphocytes, and B-ly7 is expressed by very few circulating normal or tumour cells [383]. B-ly7 recognises almost all cases of HCL, and 10–50% of HCL-V or SLVL [257]. B-ly7 expression is thus very useful in distinguishing typical HCL from 'non-hairy' disorders, but is less useful in distinguishing between HCL and HCL-V or SLVL.
HC2	++	Initially raised against HCs, the HC2 antigen is also expressed by activated normal B and T cells [300], activated (and non-activated) monocytes and mantle zone cells [214]. The antigen is not expressed by CLL, and is rarely present on HCL-V or SLVL [257]. A significant problem with this marker, however, is that 20–40% of typical HCL do not express HC2 [214], and the antibody may be less readily available.

should be recognised that no single Mab can be considered HC-specific, and all 'specific' antigens can occur on other cell types, or may individually be absent from otherwise typical cases. Table 4.3 gives a guide to HC reactivity with the most widely used diagnostic Mabs in HCL.

Finally, a number of specific HC-related conditions have been identified and their clinico-pathological features are now well characterised. These specific disorders can usually be recognised by their typical combinations of features; they are described in Section 4.4.

4.4
Variant forms of HCL and closely related conditions

Hairy-cell leukaemia variant (HCL-V) Initially described in 1980 [74], this disorder is closely related to typical HCL, but has distinct clinico-pathological features. The principal clinical characteristics of the disorder are given in Table 4.4 [74, 315].

The cytological features of the malignant cell clearly separate HCL-V from typical HCL (Plate 3 and Fig. 4.1). The malignant cell is smaller than the HC, with a higher nuclear–cytoplasmic ratio. The nucleus is centrally placed and is round or indented with clumped chromatin. A small nucleolus is present in the majority of cells and occasional binucleate cells are seen. The cytoplasm is basophilic, and hairs are less prominent than in typical HCL [69, 74].

The pathology differs significantly from that of typical HCL. Bone marrow is easily aspirated and malignant cells may be present in clumps. On trephine, an interstitial or nodular pattern of infiltration is seen and reticulin is only slightly increased. In contrast, splenic and hepatic histopathology reveal features very similar to those of typical HCL.

Surface marker expression closely resembles that of HCs with strong sIg, CD19, CD20, CD22 and FMC7 generally present. However, the disorder can generally be discriminated from typical HCL by its lack of expression of the two activation antigens, CD25 and HC2 [257]. The HC-specific integrin receptors CD11c and B-ly7 are often expressed on HCL-V (Table 4.6).

Accurate discrimination between HCL-V and typical HCL is important since variant disease has a relatively poor response to therapy. Generally the disease does

Table 4.4 Features of HCL-V

Average age	Approximately 70 years.
Sex ratio	Equal.
Blood involvement	A high leukocyte count is usually seen, typically 50–100 $\times$ 10^9/l. Marrow function is usually well preserved; monocytopenia is not a feature.
Tissue involvement	Splenic enlargement is the major presenting feature, and may be considerable. Hepatic or lymph node enlargement is not seen.
TRAP	Weak or absent.
Comment	Weight loss, fatigue and symptoms of splenic enlargement form the typical presentation. The clinical course is relatively benign with a median survival >4 years, but response to IFN or to nucleosides is poor.

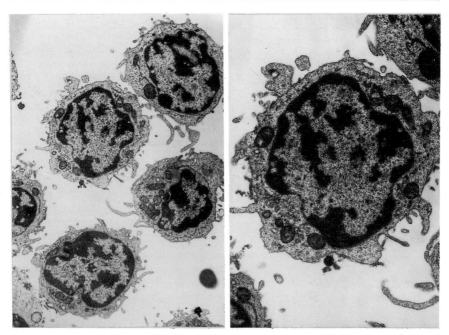

Fig. 4.1. Hairy cell variant. The high nuclear–cytoplasmic ratio and relatively heavy peripheral chromatin condensation of the cells are shown; surface hairs are relatively inconspicuous.

not respond to IFN, and the response to splenectomy is poor or absent [315, 402]. Nucleosides may be effective but usually result in only a partial response [202, 315]. Chlorambucil may have some benefit [402]. Despite this poor response to treatment, HCL-V is a relatively benign disorder and survival is generally prolonged without therapy.

Splenic lymphoma with villous lymphocytes The principal clinical features of SLVL (summarised in Table 4.5) often resemble those of typical HCL, although the presence of lymph node enlargement or a monoclonal Ig are useful indicators of SLVL [71, 260, 274]. Cytological and pathological features are more distinctive [179, 274]. The malignant cell is intermediate in size between the HC and the CLL cell. Its nucleus is round or ovoid, with condensed chromatin; a small nucleolus is usually visible. Cytoplasm is less abundant than in HCL; short villi are present, but these may be inconspicuous or confined to the poles of the malignant cell (Plate 4). Cells with plasmacytoid differentiation may occasionally be seen.

Bone marrow is easily aspirated, but malignant cells are not always identified in aspirates or biopsies. When present, marrow involvement is usually nodular or patchy, and may occasionally show a paratrabecular pattern. Splenic pathology is distinctive: malignant cells are typically confined to discrete nodules; red pulp involvement is seen and may dominate the distribution; however, white pulp involvement always occurs.

Immunophenotypic studies may assist in differentiating the condition from HCL or HCL-V. However, the immunophenotype of all three disorders may be very

Table 4.5 Features of SLVL

Average age	Approximately 70 years.
Sex ratio	Slight male predominance.
Blood involvement	Malignant cells circulate in numbers similar to those seen in typical HCL. Marrow function is often well preserved and monocytopenia is not a feature.
Tissue involvement	Splenic enlargement is seen in over 90% of cases and may be considerable. Hepatic and lymph node enlargement are less common, but are more frequent than in HCL. Bone marrow is usually easily aspirable.
TRAP	TRAP reactivity is usually present, but is generally low to moderate, occurring in only a minority of cells.
Comment	Weight loss, fatigue and symptoms of splenic enlargement form the typical presentation. Monoclonal IgM (or IgD) is often detected in plasma (60%).

similar. In common with HCL and HCL-V, the SLVL cell expresses mature/activated B-cell markers, CD19, 20, 22 and FMC7, while CD5 and CD38 are usually absent. CD11c, CD25, HC2 and B-ly7 may each be present on individual cases, but less commonly than in typical HCL. The relative frequency of these four markers has been compared in the three disorders, and the results are summarised in Table 4.6 (from [257]). The authors of that study emphasised that no single case of SLVL expressed more than two of the four markers together, whereas in typical HCL three or four markers were co-expressed in 98% of cases. Immunophenotypic discrimination between SLVL and HCL-V can be more difficult since a similar immunophenotype is often seen (Table 4.6). The present treatment of choice for SLVL is splenectomy.

Table 4.6 Surface expression of 'HC-specific' antigens in HCL and related disorders*

Surface antigen	HCL	HCL-V	SLVL
CD11c	+++	++	++
CD25	+++	±	+
HC2	++	±	±
B-ly7	+++	+	+

Source: Adapted from [257].
*Percentage of cases expressing antigen: +++, >90%; ++, 50–90%; +, 0–50%; ±, 0–10%.

Japanese form of HCL In Western countries, HCL presents a well-defined clinico-pathological entity with little variation in incidence or features between different geographical areas [338]. However, in Japan an apparently unique variant of the disease is seen, and typical HCL and HCL-V are relatively rare [365]. The Japanese form of HCL has particular morphological and haematological features that distinguish it as a distinct disorder [207].

The clinical and pathological features reported in the largest series [247] are summarised in Table 4.7. The essential clinical features closely resemble those of the Western form of the disease, although there are differences in age and sex incidence.

Table 4.7 Features of Japanese HCL

Average age	Approximately 65 years.
Sex ratio	Equal or slight female predominance.
Blood involvement	The white cell count is typically higher than in HCL, but normally lower than in HCL-V. The cells have unique features (see text), and marrow function is relatively well preserved.
Tissue involvement	Pathological appearances of bone marrow, spleen and lymph node all resemble Western disease.
TRAP	Moderate to strong reactivity is seen in most cases.
Comment	No reported cases outside Japan; response to therapy may be reduced.

The morphology and immunophenotype of the abnormal cell, however, differ significantly from those of typical HCL. Malignant cells from Japanese HCL have a round nucleus and an aggregated nuclear chromatin that contrasts with the reticular pattern of typical HCL. Cytoplasm is abundant but, while projections are clearly present on phase-contrast microscopy or scanning electron microscopy, the membrane outline on blood smears is smooth or slightly irregular (Plate 5). Immunophenotypically, the cells resemble those in the Western form of the disease in their expression of CD20, CD11c and sIg (principally IgG) and in their absence of CD5. However, in contrast to typical HCL, CD25 is generally not present and B-ly7 expression is uncommon [247].

It is unclear why an unusual form of the disease should predominate in Japan, and as yet no Western cases of the disorder have been reported. The diagnosis has prognostic implications since the disorder is less responsive to IFN than is typical HCL [247].

Monocytoid B-cell lymphoma Monocytoid B-cell lymphoma (MCBCL) was initially described in 1986 [328]. In pathological sections, MCBCL cells share with HCs certain features of distribution and immuno-reactivity. The rare circulating

Table 4.8 Features of monocytoid B-cell lymphoma

Average age	Approximately 60 years.
Sex ratio	Equal or slight male predominance.
Blood involvement	Pathological cells resemble HCs but are rare in peripheral blood, where they have been reported only in cases with advanced disease and bulky lymph nodes. Bone marrow involvement occurs late; monocytopenia is not a feature.
Tissue involvement	Principally lymph node enlargement, although MALT sites are commonly involved and such involvement may be the presenting feature. Hepatic and splenic enlargement usually occurs late, but may occasionally be seen without lymph node involvement.
TRAP	Not present.
Comment	B symptoms of lymphoma are common. Transformation to high-grade lymphoma is described [81].

monocytoid B cells may have a hairy-like morphology. However, the disorder is clinically and pathologically distinct from HCL, and the diagnostic similarities with HCL have probably been overemphasised. The typical clinical presentation and important features are given in Table 4.8 [81, 328, 367].

The pathological appearances of monocytoid B cell lymphoma have been well documented. Lymph node appearances vary, but the sinuses of the interfollicular areas are typically involved. Such extensive infiltration contrasts with that of HCL, but the cells may resemble HCs in their monomorphic appearance and abundant cytoplasm. In bone marrow trephines the malignant cells show a typical paratrabecular distribution with no fine reticulin fibrosis [329]. However, splenic appearances may resemble those of HCL, with prominent red pulp involvement (although pseudosinuses and blood lakes do not occur) [367]. Immunological reactivity on paraffin sections may also resemble that of HCL (Table 4.2) since the malignant cells react with L26 and 4KB5; however, DBA.44 reactivity is uncommon [282, 100].

Circulating MCBCL cells may occur as a late feature of the disorder, and the abnormal cells may be present in marrow aspirates. Appearances may vary greatly, but large atypical lymphoid cells with round or ovoid nuclei and abundant cytoplasm with projections may occasionally be seen. Limited immunocytochemical studies of such cells suggest certain similarities with HCL (CD5 negative, CD20 and CD11c positive, and PCA-1 variable). However, CD25 has been reported to be not expressed [329, 366] and the cells do not possess TRAP [366].

4.5
Atypical and rare presentations

In addition to the relatively well-defined hairy-like disorders, other variants have been described (Table 4.9; HCL with T-cell features; HCL/CLL; HCL/MCBCL). These

Table 4.9 Uncommon presentations of HCL

Description	Comment	References
HCL with T-cell features	Well-defined HCL/HCL-V with immunophenotype and/or molecular characteristics of T-cells.	[91, 131, 159, 285, 17]
HCL/CLL	HCL-like cases have been described with hybrid cytology/immunophenotype and clinical features intermediate between HCL and CLL.	[158, 225, 6]
HCL/MCBCL	A disorder sharing immunophenotypic and pathological features of both HCL and MCBCL.	[2]
Hypoplastic presentation of HCL	Myeloid aplasia preceding the appearance of typical HCL.	[253]
Primary splenic HCL	Malignant cells absent from blood or bone marrow.	[34, 275]
Fibrotic presentations	Myelofibrosis preceding recognisable HCL.	[162, 351]

variants share features with typical HCL, but differ significantly in one or more important aspects. Furthermore, a number of unusual presentations of otherwise typical HCL are recorded in the literature, usually as isolated cases or small series (Table 4.9; hypoplasia, splenic and fibrotic disease).

CHAPTER 5

Treatment: Mechanisms

HCL shows a poor response to conventional cytotoxic chemotherapy, but can be very effectively suppressed by a number of measures. The different therapeutic modalities are not clearly related in their action, but one general principle seems to apply. When the malignant cells are significantly reduced by any measure, HCs are slow to reappear and prolonged remission is common. When the 'cell kill' is very high, as may be seen following nucleoside analogue treatment, very prolonged remission (and perhaps cure) is seen.

Particularly with respect to nucleoside therapy, and to a lesser extent with IFN treatment, HCL has provided a model for the successful application of treatments that have subsequently been more widely applied. Perhaps for this reason, there has been considerable research interest in how the different treatments achieve their therapeutic benefit. The purpose of this chapter is to review the possible mechanisms of action of the major treatment options in HCL.

General Summary

- Splenectomy reduces peripheral pooling of normal haemic cells and, by 'debulking' effects, may reduce HC-derived suppressive and autoproliferative factors.
- αIFN and βIFN act directly on HCs and also on other immune cells. Their therapeutic benefit appears to result from a direct inhibition of HC proliferation, probably as a result of an alteration in the state of activation or differentiation of the malignant cell.
- CDA, deoxycoformycin (DCF) and fludarabine function as analogues of 2′-deoxyadenosine and cause an abnormal accumulation of products in the deoxycytidine kinase pathway. Their exact mechanism of action is unclear, but does not require cell division. Inhibition of DNA repair, disturbed RNA metabolism, metabolic exhaustion and disturbed transmethylation have all been described. The mode of HC death is apoptosis.

5.1
Mechanism of action of splenectomy

It has been repeatedly reported that there is significant pooling of blood cells within the spleen [188, 250]. It has been proposed, therefore, that the principal mechanism underlying the response of HCL to splenectomy is a reduction of splenic pooling. In this regard, splenectomy is effective principally in patients in whom marrow reserve is good, and ineffective where severe marrow suppression exists [305].

However, the effectiveness of splenectomy is largely, although not entirely, independent of spleen size [138, 305]. Furthermore, while in most cases the response to the procedure is limited, there are undoubted cases of disease regression and very long remission following the procedure [35, 73]. Other mechanisms for the beneficial effect of splenectomy may therefore exist. In this regard there is limited, but accumulating, evidence that the spleen may be a proliferative site or an area where HCs are relatively protected by microenvironmental interactions from the damaging effects of chemotherapy [286, 353]. Furthermore, it is now recognised that secreted factors from HCs exert a strong suppressive effect on normal marrow elements [112, 355]. It seems likely, therefore, that splenic 'debulking' may act both to remove an important area of HC proliferation and to reduce suppression of normal marrow cells.

5.2
The mechanism of action of αIFN

IFN-induced effects on HCs are divisible into 'direct' effects against the HC itself, and 'indirect' effects that are mediated through the action of other immune cells.

5.2.1
Indirect effects

A profound disturbance of immune cell function is consistently found in HCL. Monocytopenia is characteristic [325, 376], T-cell subsets are disordered [357, 358, 374, 376], and both B [277] and NK cells [92, 278, 374] are reduced in number and have altered function. This depressed immunity is probably multifactorial in origin. Factors that may be important include marrow infiltration/fibrosis [223, 360], reduced levels of stimulatory cytokines [121] and the secretion of inhibitory factors by malignant HCs [224, 355]. In addition to this suppression of immune effector cells, the HC itself presents a poor target for immune destruction by NK cells [83, 147, 340] or by cytotoxic T cells [324]. This poor immune recognition stems at least partly from the low expression by HCs of MHC antigens [119, 145] and of functionally associated molecules such as LFA-1 [193].

These observations might suggest that the impaired immune cell function in HCL and the failure of immune cells to recognise HCs together allow unopposed expansion of the malignant clone. By extension, the beneficial effects of IFN might be the result of IFN-induced 'regeneration' of the immune response. These possibilities are not, however, supported by present data.

It is clear that immune function is improved during IFN therapy. For example, bone marrow function is restored [224], fibrosis may regress [360], NK-cell and T-cell function and number are restored [84, 193, 374, 387] and immune recognition of HCs may be enhanced through IFN-induced upregulation of MHC and LFA-1 [119, 145, 193]. However, there is no clear evidence to support the view that this improved immune function underlies the therapeutic response to IFN [380]. HCs are resistant to killing *in vitro* by NK or LAK cells derived from IFN-treated patients [84, 147, 340]. Moreover, IFN-induced changes in immune cell constitution do not precede the reduction of HC tumour load [277]. Present evidence therefore suggests that the immune recovery is a secondary phenomenon resulting from, rather than causing, the HC destruction [380].

5.2.2
'Direct' anti-proliferative activity

Autocrine proliferation loops have been demonstrated for both B-cell growth factor (BCGF) and TNFα (Sections 7.7.1 and 7.7.2). Both of these cytokines have been implicated in the effects of IFN.

In the case of BCGF, the induced proliferation is inhibited by αIFN, but not by γIFN [119, 266]. Proposed mechanisms include the inhibition of the BCGF signalling pathway [125, 126] and the alteration of HC activation/differentiation [119]. As yet, the precise mechanism has not been established.

TNFα at high concentration induces HC proliferation. Like the BCGF effect, this TNFα-induced proliferation is inhibited by αIFN [28]. Heslop et al. showed that the half life of TNFα mRNA is shortened following αIFN treatment in vitro, probably as a result of mRNA destruction by IFN-induced 2-5A synthetase [167]. They postulated that TNFα secretion might be reduced by αIFN and that inhibition of the autocrine proliferation loop might thereby result [168]. In accordance with this theory, in vivo studies have demonstrated that serum TNFα levels are reduced following successful IFN treatment [112].

However, studies on HCs in vitro have shown that αIFN increases rather than reduces rates of TNFα secretion, perhaps by increasing TNFα mRNA translation [195]. These in vitro concepts have received support from in vivo studies that have identified raised serum levels of TNFα in the early phases of αIFN treatment [30, 31]. Indeed, it has been suggested that at the relatively low levels of TNFα found in blood and bone marrow aspirates, the cytokine acts to inhibit rather than enhance HC proliferation. αIFN may therefore act to increase this suppression by stimulating further TNF production [31].

These apparently conflicting ideas may not be incompatible. The precise kinetics of TNF secretion by HCs has not been established [169]. Moreover, it is now recognised that TNFα binds to high- and low-affinity receptors, which mediate different signals and functional responses [19, 170]. As described in Section 7.7.2, both forms of TNF receptor may be expressed by HCs under different conditions [30, 371]. Thus, TNFα may induce different signals in HCs within different tissue compartments according to local cytokine concentration and HC receptor expression.

5.2.3
Modification of intracellular signals by αIFN

There is increasing evidence that the outward manifestations of cell activation that characterise the malignant HC are a consequence of 'intracellular' activation. Manifestations of this activation include the demonstration that HCs, as compared with normal and related malignant B-cell populations, display the following: elevated levels of intracytoplasmic free calcium [130]; increased activity of serine/threonine kinases/phosphatases and tyrosine-protein kinases/phosphatases [186, 244, 246]; and enhanced phosphorylation of membrane signalling molecules such as CD20 [129]. Attention has therefore focused on how IFN might modify HC signalling processes.

In other cell types, binding of IFN to its specific receptor induces rapid activation of tyrosine kinase signalling cascades, resulting in alterations in intracellular and membrane phosphorylation. Such changes precede the activation of specific intracytoplasmic and nuclear effector molecules that alter proliferation and differentiation (reviewed in [288]). Investigation of IFN-induced changes in the cell signalling activity of HCs has suggested analogous changes. Genot and Wietzerbin have shown that αIFN reduces intracellular free calcium levels within HCs, and decreases the phosphorylation of CD20 and perhaps of other signalling molecules within the cell (reviewed in [130]). Although proto-oncogene activity in HCs (e.g. raf-1 [354], c-myc and c-fos [229]) has not been linked to IFN sensitivity, evidence has recently been presented that in the HC-derived cell line ESKOL, certain proto-oncogenes involved in B-cell activation/differentiation are downregulated by IFN [160].

5.2.4
Altered differentiation/activation state

Altered signalling resulting from IFN exposure may directly reduce HC proliferation. However, the IFN effect is also reflected in characteristic changes in cell surface antigen expression and cytoskeletal organisation. Such changes are widely believed to signify an alteration in the state of differentiation or activation of the malignant cell.

IFN-induced changes in cell morphology, reflecting membrane and cytoskeletal alterations, have been described repeatedly. The characteristic surface villi of the HC are reduced in number [251] and altered in form, becoming more broad based and blunt [118, 268]. The spectrin content of the cells is reduced [103]. TRAP expression is lower [161] and, at an ultrastructural level, a reduction in ribosome–lamellar (R–L) complexes and an increase in tubulo-reticular structures have been reported [268].

Pronounced alterations were also seen at the cell surface. Surface Ig expression, the IL-2 receptor α chain (CD25), FMC7, CD71 and, in some reports, the β2 integrin p150,95 (CD11c) are all reduced [119, 161, 251, 361]. Expression of MHC antigens, the β2 integrin LFA-1 (CD11a) and CD22 are increased.

How the various changes described above contribute to the anti-proliferative effects of IFN is not clear. Inhibition of autocrine proliferation is unlikely to be the sole mediator of the IFN effect. However, altered production of autocrine factors together with altered cell signalling and changes in membrane receptor engagement are all likely to be important. Such alterations will affect the interaction of the HC with its microenvironment at all levels (cytokine interaction, adhesion and migration, and cell–cell contact). Thus, αIFN-induced changes in HC biology may be viewed as an 'altered state of differentiation', the net effect of which may be to change the capacity of the HC to receive important proliferative signals from its microenvironment.

5.3
Mechanism of action of the purine analogue drugs

All three of these agents (CDA. DCF and fludarabine) act primarily to disrupt the normal salvage pathways for purine nucleosides. The exact mechanism by which the drugs mediate their beneficial effect in HCL has not been established. However, the basic mechanisms that may underlie the activity of the drugs appear similar and are therefore considered together.

5.3.1
Normal purine metabolism in lymphoid cells: the role of adenosine deaminase

The peculiar sensitivity of lymphocytes to purine analogue drugs results from the use within lymphoid tissues of particular salvage pathways for purine nucleosides (reviewed in [60]). In lymphocytes, purine nucleosides, including deoxyadenosine, undergo salvage metabolism in which the rate-limiting enzyme is deoxycytidine kinase (dCK). The action of this enzyme is to generate deoxynucleoside triphosphates (dNTPs) that are available for incorporation into DNA. Appreciable dCK activity is present even in resting lymphocytes. It is thought that this activity generates a small pool of dNTPs, which is utilised in DNA repair or in the rapid synthesis of DNA required following antigen stimulation.

However, when DNA catabolism occurs or when deoxyadenosine is present at high levels within the circulation, dCK has the potential to produce high levels of deoxyadenosine triphosphate within the lymphocytes. Protection from such toxic accumulation is provided by the enzyme adenosine deaminase (ADA). ADA is highly expressed in lymphoid tissue and rapidly deaminates any excess deoxyadenosine, forming the non-toxic product deoxyinosine (Fig. 5.1).

Such ADA-mediated degradation of deoxyadenosine appears to be vital for lymphocyte survival. The rare congenital deficiency of ADA results in a severe combined immunodeficiency with drastically reduced numbers of lymphoid cells. In this congenital condition, high levels of dATP are thought to mediate the specific destruction of lymphoid cells. Other cell types are relatively spared because they do

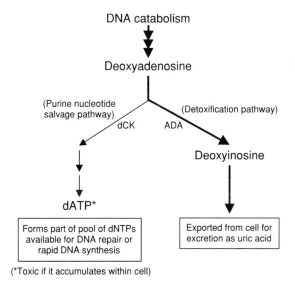

Fig 5.1. The two principal routes of metabolism of deoxyadenosine within lymphoid cells.

not employ the nucleotide salvage pathway and do not, therefore, generate high levels of dATP.

5.3.2
Adenosine deaminase function in the presence of purine analogue drugs

The three drugs, DCF, CDA and fludarabine are all analogues of 2'-deoxyadenosine (Fig. 5.2). They mediate their primary effects through the pathway of the enzyme ADA.

DCF mimics a transition state during the deamination of deoxyadenosine and acts as a tight-binding reversible inhibitor of ADA. DCF therefore causes an accumulation of dATP [41].

CDA and fludarabine are halogen substituted analogues of deoxyadenosine that are highly resistant to deamination by ADA but are readily phosphorylated by dCK. Administration of CDA or fludarabine therefore leads to the accumulation of the triphosphate form of the drug itself [42, 312]. In this review the triphosphate forms of these drugs or of deoxyadenosine itself are collectively referred to as deoxynucleoside triphosphates (dNTPs).

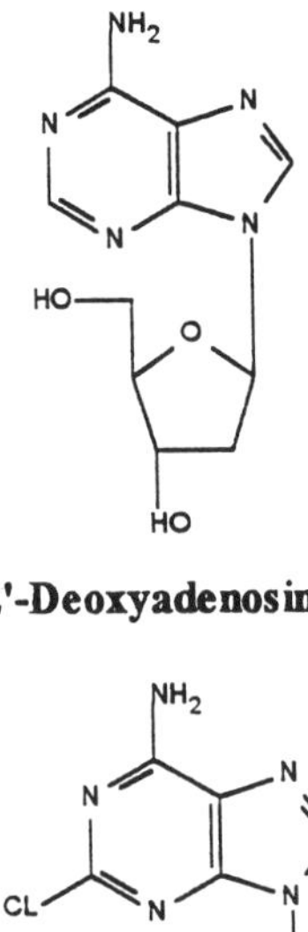

2'-Deoxyadenosine 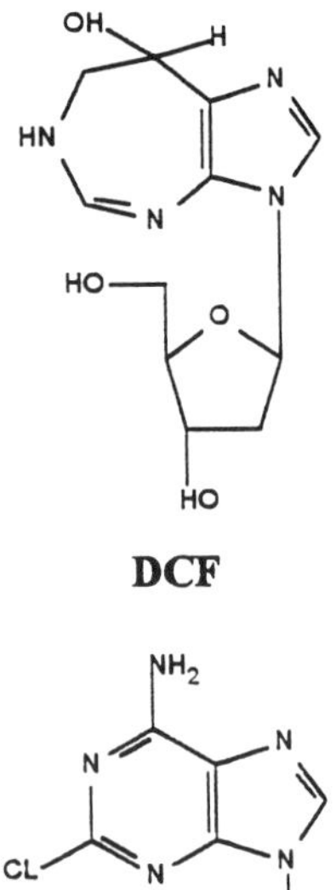   **DCF**

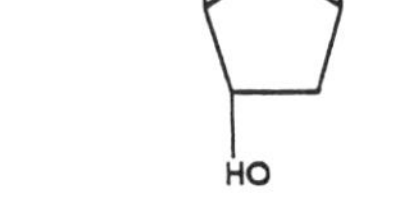

CDA 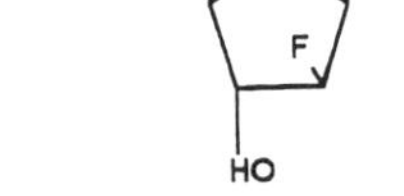   **Fludarabine**

Fig. 5.2. Deoxyadenosine and the purine analogue drugs. Note that for the prodrug fludarabine the active intracellular form is illustrated.

5.3.3
Action of purine analogue drugs on malignant cells

A number of potential mechanisms by which dNTPs may induce toxicity have been proposed. Toxic effects related to cell division can clearly occur, and are described in the following subsection. However, purine analogues differ from most chemotherapeutic agents in their ability to mediate toxicity against non-dividing cells [61]; this is likely to be of particular importance in slowly dividing cells such as HCs, and is considered in the later subsections.

Mechanisms of action in rapidly dividing cells The accumulation of dNTPs is toxic to dividing cells. All three drugs cause allosteric inhibition of ribonucleotide reductase, resulting in depletion of the normal deoxynucleotides; this lack of normal nucleotides inhibits effective DNA synthesis [41, 42, 312]. In addition, the triphosphate forms of CDA and fludarabine may be incorporated into DNA, where they may inhibit chain extension [42].

Mechanisms of action in slowly dividing cells The precise mechanism by which the purine analogue drugs achieve their clinical efficacy in slowly dividing lymphoid cells such as HCs is not known. However, it is clear that the purine analogues induce a number of effects not directly related to cell division. These mechanisms, together or independently, may contribute to the toxic effects of the nucleoside drugs.

Disturbance of DNA repair Lymphocytes naturally form single and repeat DNA strand breaks. When the cells are treated with purine analogues, such single strand breaks accumulate [82], possibly through the action of endonucleases activated by the imbalance in dNTP levels [171]. The repair of natural DNA damage requires the binding of poly(ADP-ribose) to the damaged area. Abnormal accumulation of dNTPs inhibits natural DNA repair and this leads to an increased requirement for poly(ADP-ribose). The required formation of large amounts of poly(ADP-ribose) by the affected cell consumes cell NAD+ and ATP and can lead to cell death through metabolic exhaustion [326].

Disruption of normal RNA balance RNA synthesis may be reduced by purine nucleoside analogues through the inhibition of transcriptional activity [256]. Furthermore, breakdown of short-chain mRNA may be enhanced through nucleoside-induced transcription of 2-5 A synthetase [120, 176]. The net effect is to disrupt the biosynthesis of essential proteins/peptides.

Disordered transmethylation reactions Transmethylation reactions are important in the control of gene transcription and of other cell processes. Purine nucleotide analogues inhibit the enzyme S-adenosyl homocysteine hydrolase (SAH). By inhibiting catabolism of SAH, the drugs disturb the normal balance between SAH and its precursor S-adenosylmethionine (SAM). As a result, transmethylation reactions in which SAM is the methyl donor are inhibited [173]. It has been suggested that SAH hydrolase levels correlate well with clinical response [173], but a subsequent report from the same group failed to confirm this correlation [174].

Apoptosis and purine analogues Although the precise biochemical mechanisms underlying the toxicity of the nucleosides is not clear, it is accepted that the outcome for the affected cell is to undergo 'programmed cell death' (apoptosis) [61, 256]. This has been shown both in CLL cells, where apoptotic responses to therapy are well documented [61], and also in HCL [173]. This nucleoside-induced apoptotic cell death clearly distinguishes the effects of these drugs from the anti-proliferative/ differentiating effects of IFN.

Mechanism of action in hairy cells It is clear that the nucleosides have therapeutic activity against a range of lymphoid malignancies. However, the pronounced sensitivity of typical HCL to the drugs is unexplained. Several studies have examined the role of the specific mechanisms discussed above in relation to HCL. It has not been possible, however, to correlate the known *in vitro* effects of the drugs with clinical responses to such therapy. In a large study of the clinical response of HCL to treatment with DCF, Ho et al. showed no significant correlation between outcome and DNA strand break formation, NAD+ levels, ATP levels or SAH hydrolase activity [174].

In an alternative approach, Ganashaguru et al. examined the effects of the nucleosides on the endonuclease 2-5A synthetase, which has been implicated in the clinical response of HCs to IFN (Section 5.2.2) [120]. 2-5A synthetase was shown to be rapidly induced in HCL cases responding to DCF, but not in non-responsive cases. The significance of these observations is, however, unclear. It is difficult to envisage that IFN and the nucleosides share a common pathway of action given the different responses of HCL to the two types of treatment. Moreover, it is not clear whether the 2-5A synthetase was induced in the HCs or in accompanying T cells.

Finally, it has been reported that DCF renders HCs more susceptible to killing by NK cells [222]. Whether this is a specific effect of the drug on NK cells or whether the susceptibility of HCs to killing is a reflection of drug-induced apoptosis has not been established. At present, therefore, it must be concluded that the specific mechanism(s) of action of these drugs in HCL is yet to be established.

CHAPTER 6

Treatment: Practical Considerations

General summary

- The nucleoside analogue drugs CDA and DCF are now established as the treatment of choice in HCL.

- Over 90% of cases respond to treatment with nucleoside analogues, and 'complete remission' is induced in over 75% of cases. Present evidence suggests that most patients will have a prolonged disease-free survival following nucleoside treatment.

- IFN and splenectomy remain effective treatments for HCL and retain a place in the treatment of relapsed disease and in certain specific clinical circumstances.

- The place of growth factors in the treatment of HCL is unclear, but they have been shown to improve neutrophil counts and help resolve infections before therapy or during IFN treatment. No benefit has yet been demonstrated for growth factors given in conjunction with nucleosides.

6.1
When should treatment be commenced?

Significant debility or infection is uncommon in HCL while peripheral blood values of haemoglobin, neutrophils and platelets are normal. Moreover, the disease may remain stable for prolonged periods, or occasionally may undergo spontaneous remission of prolonged duration [35, 73].

Since all present treatment strategies potentially cause morbidity, and in some cases mortality, it seems appropriate to delay specific therapy until there is significant risk of debility. Criteria for commencing treatment were proposed at the 2nd International Workshop on HCL in1986 [70] and are given in Table 6.1.

Although these criteria were defined before the widespread use of purine analogues (nucleosides), it is likely that they will continue to be employed as reasonable guidelines. Treatment with these agents is so effective that the aim of therapy is now prolonged disease-free remission with effective or actual cure. The nucleosides are best tolerated when marrow suppression is minimal. There may

Table 6.1. Criteria for commencing therapy in HCL

Onset of recurrent or serious infections
Granulocyte count unstable or less than $1.5 \times 10^9/l$
Significant anaemia (<12 g/dl) or transfusions required
Bleeding tendency or platelets <100 $\times$ $10^9/l$

therefore be an increasing desire on the part of both patient and physician to commence therapy earlier.

Although the nucleosides are now the mainstay of treatment, splenectomy and αIFN have in the past proved effective treatments and are likely to retain some role in the disease. These two treatment options will be considered before moving on to the purine analogues. The chapter ends with a short section on the colony-stimulating factors.

6.2
Splenectomy

Summary

- The procedure is well tolerated and, among current therapeutic options, offers the most rapid improvement in platelet count.
- The overall response rate is between 70 and 90%, but only 40–60% of these will achieve a normal or near normal blood count. Prolonged responses may be seen in up to 10%, but loss of response is usual and the mean time to treatment failure is 19 months.
- Although splenectomy can no longer be recommended as primary treatment in most individuals, it may retain a place for 'splenic HCL', for patients with severe bleeding and where patients wish to avoid systemic therapy.

Practical considerations

Morbidity/mortality: No specific problems related to HCL. Mortality and morbidity probably similar to that for splenectomy in other lymphoproliferative disorders (1–5% and 30%, respectively).

Precautions: Pneumococcal vaccine/antibiotic prophylaxis according to local splenectomy policy.

Contraindications (relative): Small spleen, extensive marrow suppression, current infection, poor surgical risk.

Response: Rapid platelet response (days) with possible overshoot, neutrophil response may be poor.

6.2.1
Therapeutic value of splenectomy

Outcome of splenectomy Comparison of studies is difficult since patient selection and measures of outcome differ between centres. However, the outcome of a number of large studies suggests that between 70 and 90% of patients will show haematological improvement following splenectomy [189]. Between 40 and 60% will achieve a normal or near normal peripheral blood count [35]. Although the mean time to treatment failure is 19 months, patients with good bone marrow reserve have a failure-free survival of 4.5 years [304]. In those patients with the 'splenic form' of HCL where there is little or no bone marrow involvement, splenectomy may be curative [35].

The procedure has a low risk of mortality [196], and the overall 5-year survival following splenectomy is around 70% [138]. This is a significant survival advantage over unsplenectomised subjects; in one series of 105 patients, splenectomy allowed an average survival of 6.9 years compared with 4.8 years in unsplenectomised subjects [35].

It is clear, however, that a proportion of patients derive no survival benefit from splenectomy. To identify those patients most likely to benefit from splenectomy, therefore, a number of staging systems have been developed (Section 2.3). The most widely used system was developed by Jansen and Hermans on the basis of a multicentre analysis of prognostic variables [190]. With regard to pre-splenectomy features, essentially any patient with a spleen palpable 4 cm below the costal margin, or with a palpable spleen and anaemia will benefit from surgery. A subsequent study by Golomb and Vardiman emphasised that extensive bone marrow involvement is a predictor of poor response to spleen removal [138].

Present role of splenectomy When compared with newer treatments, splenectomy provides a relatively low incidence and duration of remission and, although the procedure is relatively safe, there remains a potential for operative morbidity or mortality [196]. It has been formally shown that splenectomy is less effective than αIFN in inducing haematological remission [56, 332]. Splenectomy cannot therefore be regarded as first-line therapy in most cases of HCL. Removal of the spleen of patients responding to IFN does not prolong their survival [107] and is not popular with patients [87].

However, prolonged clinical responses to splenectomy may occur, and the treatment avoids the use of systemic chemotherapeutic drugs. Compared with other treatments, splenectomy offers the most rapid improvement in platelet count [35, 332], and prior splenectomy does not reduce the effectiveness of other treatments.

Splenectomy may therefore offer advantages to certain patients. In particular, this form of therapy may be appropriate for those patients wishing to avoid systemic therapy (especially those with splenic HCL or with good bone marrow reserve), or where a rapid platelet response is the primary requirement.

There are no data on the effectiveness of splenectomy in the treatment of patients resistant to the newer systemic treatments. However, because the mechanism underlying the beneficial effect of splenectomy must differ from that of the nucleosides, it seems reasonable to predict that patients resistant to nucleosides might respond to splenectomy.

6.3
Interferon

Summary

- Treatment with αIFN induces a normal blood count in around 80% of patients, but only around 10% achieve an apparently normal marrow. Relapse after stopping IFN is usual, and further treatment is generally required after a mean of 2–3 years. However, around 20% require no further treatment 5 years after initial therapy. Long-term treatment appears to offer certain benefits.
- IFN is well tolerated in HCL and causes less marrow suppression than newer

agents. However, minor side effects are common and fatigue may be debilitating. Such effects can be minimised by the use of maintenance regimes.

- IFN can no longer be considered as a primary therapeutic agent in HCL, but may retain a role as second-line treatment or where marrow suppression is severe.

Practical considerations

Therapeutic dose: Varies; 2×10^6 U/m^2/day for 4–6 months, then three times weekly until one year; low-dose or maintenance regimes may be useful in some individuals.

Mortality: Early mortality relates to disease activity/infection; late deaths from second malignancy are now reported.

Side effects: Major side effects are neurotoxicity and autoimmune disease (rare); minor side effects are common and include 'flu-like' symptoms and fatigue.

Speed of response: Therapeutic benefit is usually apparent within 2 months and normal blood counts may occur after 3–5 months; continued improvement may be seen throughout treatment.

Follow-up: Extensive marrow involvement, thrombocytopenia or high NAP score after completion of IFN may predict early peripheral blood relapse.

6.3.1
Therapeutic activity of IFN in HCL

The advent of more effective therapy for HCL in the form of DCF and 2CDA has reduced the clinical role of αIFN as primary treatment. However, the low toxicity of IFN, the wealth of clinical experience with its use and the lack of cross resistance between IFN and the nucleosides mean that IFN is likely to retain a place in HCL therapy for quite some time.

Clinical trials have repeatedly confirmed that αIFN has a clear beneficial effect in most cases of HCL, and in some instances induces prolonged clinical remission. This section attempts to provide an overview of IFN therapy. Initially, 'standard' therapy is considered (that is, 2–3 × 10^{6}U/day for 4–6 months followed by 2 or 3 × 10^{6}U three times per week for a further 6–12 months). Various problems associated with αIFN in HCL and alternative strategies for the cytokine are then considered.

Induction of remission IFN trials generally distinguish 'complete remission' (CR), where HCs constitute less than 5% of bone marrow cells, partial remission (PR), where bone marrow clearance is not achieved but peripheral counts are normalised, and patients who show minimal or no response to IFN. In 1993, Jaiyesimi et al. reviewed the 10 major reported trials involving a total of 417 patients [182]. These trials, though not strictly comparable, revealed overall response rates of CR 8%, PR 74% and minor/nil response 15% [182]. CR rates reported in recent trials are generally lower than in earlier studies. For example, a more recent trial reported by Golomb et al. [139] found a CR rate of only 4%, and a study by Berman et al. found no true CR in their cohort [24]. These apparently lower response rates probably reflect the adoption of more rigorous definitions of CR.

The prognostic significance in HCL of CR or PR is, however, far from clear. HCs are detectable in the bone marrow by immunohistology following all forms of therapy [290], and may be present in spleen during apparent bone marrow remission [286]. Furthermore, patients having initial PR may have prolonged symptom-free survival [63]. Berman et al. reported that the number of residual bone marrow hairy cells on completion of therapy had no statistical association with disease progression [24].

Duration of remission Although 80% of patients initially achieve normal peripheral bloods counts following IFN therapy, the majority of patients will eventually require further treatment. Two separate measures of disease progression have been used and are of rather different significance. The first measure is the interval between treatment and reappearance of significant disease; this is often short. The second measure is the interval between initial treatment and the requirement for further therapy, and this may be relatively long.

Berman et al. [24] have reviewed data from their own series and two comparable series. In responding patients, the time from completion of therapy to significant deterioration in peripheral counts or to reappearance of circulating HCs ranged from 6 to 10 months (n = 76). Moreover, these authors emphasised that half the patients who relapse after stopping IFN will do so within one year. However, simple 'relapse' may not require immediate treatment; the time interval between completion of therapy and the requirement for re-treatment is around 30 months [141, 304].

Survival Meaningful analysis of both early and late deaths in IFN-treated patients is now possible. Two groups have followed patients for a mean period of 5 and 6 years, respectively; in both studies, survival at 5 years was 86–87% [63, 141]. In both series, the major cause of mortality was infection, either during initial therapy or during relapse.

Interestingly, both series reported deaths from second malignancy. Although the association between HCL and second malignancy is well known (Section 2.1.2) [181], it is now clear that this association also extends to patients successfully treated with IFN [63], although a strong relationship has not been seen in all trials [115]. Thus, second malignancy developed in 15 of 69 patients followed for between 6 and 9 years [201]. In six cases, the malignancy was haematological (four non-Hodgkin's lymphoma (NHL), one acute myeloid leukaemia (AML), one histiocytosis); this excess of haematological malignancy is highly significant (observed/expected ratio 40). Clearly, second malignancy represents a major cause of death in IFN-treated HCL patients and, if seen with newer treatments, second malignancy may become the major factor determining prognosis in HCL.

Predictive factors No clear feature of HCL seems to predict the outcome of IFN therapy. At presentation, no clinical or pathological features have been identified that affect the ability of IFN to induce remission [24, 141]. Certain features have been reported to indicate a high probability of early relapse; these include extensive infiltration of bone marrow at presentation or after completion of therapy [404], a high NAP score and a low platelet count [24, 304]. However, different studies have often reached conflicting conclusions (e.g. [24, 404]).

6.3.2
Problems with IFN therapy

Toxicity and patient tolerance The side effects and toxicity of IFN have been well described (e.g. [117]). Standard doses induce initial 'flu like' symptoms in around 75% of patients; in the majority, these symptoms resolve after the first few weeks of treatment [24]. Such symptoms are well tolerated and respond to paracetamol or to night-time administration of the cytokine. More severe side effects involve the central nervous system [151] and exacerbation of autoimmune processes [151]. Both of these side effects have necessitated withdrawal of patients from major trials [141, 302]. However, treatment withdrawals due to toxicity or patient refusal are uncommon, e.g. 4 out of 69 in one major trial [141].

Resistance to IFN Between 5 and 15% of patients appear to have primary resistance to IFN and show no clinical response to initial treatment. A further group responds to the cytokine initially, but then, either as a result of antibody formation or of some other form of resistance, becomes unresponsive. Other patients are resistant to reinduction [304, 404]; such resistance is increasingly common after a second course of IFN [57]. At least two distinct mechanisms appear to apply.

Mechanisms not mediated by antibodies are responsible for most primary non-responders and for a proportion of those patients who become resistant during therapy [4]. Precise mechanisms are not clear, although lack of IFN receptor expression [296], abnormal receptor function [29] or post-receptor signalling defects [284] may all contribute.

Antibody-mediated resistance to IFN has been recognised since 1981. However, there has been considerable debate concerning both the occurrence and the significance of IFN antibodies during treatment. Important principles have now been established.

Non-neutralising antibodies detected by immunoassay but not active in viral killing (neutralising) assays may partly modify IFN pharmokinetics, but are not clinically significant [13]. In contrast, antibodies that neutralise IFN activity in functional assays have been clearly linked to loss of clinical responsiveness [345, 386]. Neutralising antibodies are probably the most important cause of secondary resistance to IFN in HCL [345].

The incidence of neutralising antibodies varies between studies. Although multiple factors may contribute [385], the differing immunogenicity of the different IFN preparations appears to be the main determinant. In separate studies of HCL, IFNα2a [345] was shown to induce a higher incidence of neutralising antibodies than IFNα2b [335, 385]. Both recombinant forms of IFN are more immunogenic than natural IFN [116]. These observations are probably in accord with the incidence of antibody formation in other disorders treated with αIFN. In a recent review, the incidence of neutralising antibody formation was IFNα2a 20%, IFNα2b 7% and nIFN 1.2% [13].

The occurrence of antibodies in a given patient does not, however, necessarily preclude further response to IFN. In many cases the antibody response is short lived, and a good clinical outcome may still be achieved by adjustment of dose or duration of therapy [346]. Furthermore, antibody cross reactivity with other IFN subtypes is low [13], and substitution of an alternative IFN preparation is usually effective [386].

6.3.3
Alternative strategies

A number of recent studies have attempted to improve the results of αIFN treatment by the use of alternative regimes.

Reduced-dose regimes Patient intolerance of IFN only rarely requires treatment withdrawal in HCL. However, dose-dependent suppression of myelopoiesis [255] may lead to problems when cytopenias are severe at the outset of treatment. Low-dose and very low-dose regimes have therefore been examined.

Low dose Doses of 1–2 MU of IFN are effective in HCL, and response rates at completion of treatment are similar to those of standard-dose regimes [163, 210, 301, 403]. Low-dose treatment may be associated with reduced side effects [403], but the rate of response may be slower [163, 210].

Very low dose Doses in the range 0.2–0.6 MU can induce remission, and have a very low incidence of side effects [123, 331]. However, very low-dose regimes are less effective than standard regimes (IFN2b [267], IFN 2c [123], nIFN [331]). Some studies have suggested that effectiveness may be improved by extending the duration of treatment [163, 279] or by tailoring the dose according to response [122].

Maintenance treatment The high relapse rate of HCL after completion of IFN therapy can be reduced by the use of maintenance IFN treatment [140, 210, 279 333]. Moreover, continued therapy for periods of up to 5 years may result in further clinical improvement [163, 279, 317, 333]. However, although major toxicity has not been seen [140, 333], minor side effects such as fatigue are common [140], and the patient withdrawal rate may approach 40% after 2 years.

Long-term treatment may be made more acceptable by the use of low-dose maintenance such as 0.5–2 MU given once or twice weekly [163, 279]. However, present evidence suggests that relapse rates on discontinuing the therapy are similar to those seen after standard therapy [139]. It seems reasonable to include maintenance therapy for any patients in whom IFN is considered appropriate treatment [57].

Other forms of IFN Type I IFNs (αIFN and βIFN) signal through the same receptor, and limited studies confirm that βIFN closely resembles αIFN in its *in vitro* effects [236, 237]. In clinical trials, βIFN has activity against HCL [133, 237, 392]. However, it does not appear to offer any therapeutic advantage and at present is not licensed for the treatment of HCL.

Type II IFN (γIFN) signals through a separate receptor also expressed on the HCs of most patients [390]. However, although αIFN and γIFN share many direct and indirect *in vitro* effects [84, 146, 266], the two agents also differ in certain important respects. For example, γIFN often has no anti-proliferative effect on HCs stimulated to divide [276]. γIFN probably has little or no therapeutic role in HCL.

IFN and splenectomy The eventual response rate and duration of remission in response to IFN therapy are unaffected by prior splenectomy [87, 109, 279, 301]. However, recovery from cytopenias appears to be more rapid in previously splenectomised patients. Moreover, after bone marrow relapse such patients may maintain their peripheral blood counts better than do non-splenectomised patients after bone marrow relapse [373].

IFN and DCF In vitro studies examining combination treatment with αIFN and DCF have identified both synergistic and antagonistic effects [222, 372]. A phase-one trial has employed the two drugs simultaneously with therapeutic benefit, and a separate trial examined the use of alternating cycles of DCF and IFN. In this latter trial (n = 15) a 100% response rate was reported, and no patient had disease progression after 27 months of follow up. However, no large studies of combination therapy have been reported.

An alternative approach has been investigated by Habermann et al. [152]. They employed standard-dose IFN administered for 3 months prior to giving DCF. The rationale behind the approach was to restore peripheral counts before commencing DCF, thereby reducing toxicity. This study suggested that the combination was as effective as DCF alone, but that infection rates were significantly reduced compared with their own historical control group treated by DCF alone. The initial use of IFN followed by DCF does seem a plausible approach in very cytopenic patients, but it should be noted that the historical controls in Haberman's study received a higher dose of DCF than did the trial patients.

6.4
Purine analogue drugs: DCF, CDA and fludarabine

Summary

- The response rate to CDA and DCF is over 90%, with 75–85% achieving apparent bone marrow remission. Sensitive techniques suggest that in many cases some residual HCs are present, but the relapse rate is low and is less than that following IFN.
- Both CDA and DCF are generally well tolerated, but neutropenia may be a problem where there is pre-existing marrow suppression.
- CDA and DCF must now be considered the principal treatments for HCL. No direct trials have compared the two agents. There is a perception that CDA is the agent of choice but, overall, the two drugs are probably comparable. More extensive experience and follow-up data exist for DCF; however, CDA may be better tolerated and perhaps offers marginally superior efficacy.

6.4.1
Therapeutic activity of DCF

Practical considerations

Dose regime: 4 mg/m^2 by intravenous (IV) bolus given every 14 days until maximum response. If remission is obtained, it is standard practice to give one or two more doses.

Mortality: Neutropenic infections are the major cause of death; neutropenia relates to marrow reserve at onset of therapy.

Side effects: Major effect is neutropenia; prolonged lymphopenia occurs but appears well tolerated; skin rashes (often photosensitive) are common; major DCF-induced renal or CNS toxicity are very uncommon at this dose; minor effects commonly include nausea and vomiting; less common are fatigue, malaise, headache, depression and transient hepatic or renal dysfunction; rare, but serious, cardiac arrhythmias/myopathy have been reported.

Response: Initial response is rapid, median time to full response being 4–7 months.

Follow up: Marrow biopsy to look for residual disease, but results are not clearly related to relapse.

Background DCF is effective therapy, both in previously untreated HCL and in patients who have relapsed following splenectomy or IFN treatment [175, 219]. The response to DCF is more rapid and more prolonged than the response to IFN [303].

Administration Current treatment protocols use a fixed, relatively low dose in the initial treatment; this is repeated at intervals until no further benefit is seen. A dose of 4 mg/m^2 is administered on alternate weeks until the blood count and bone marrow biopsy indicate that a maximal response has been attained [41, 294]. This protocol appears to offer significant advantages over earlier regimes, both in terms of effectiveness and in the incidence of side effects [12, 72]. The data presented below concerning response to therapy refer as far as possible to patients treated in this way.

Remission induction Reported response rates suggest that around 90% of patients will achieve a normal peripheral count after DCF and, of these, 74–77% will have a histological complete remission [12, 72]. Although HCs are not completely eradicated from bone marrow by DCF [359], the clearance is greater than that seen with IFNα. An improvement in clinical parameters may be expected after two cycles (4 weeks), but the median time to maximal response is approximately 4–7 months [12, 175, 219, 220].

Although patients previously treated with IFNα who have relapsed following an initial complete or partial remission respond well to DCF [175], patients primarily resistant to αIFN may respond poorly to the drug and response rates of around 35% have been reported [72].

Length of remission It is not yet possible to determine the duration of remission in response to DCF since most treatment series have run for less than 5 years. However, both CR and PR appear to be well maintained, with 77–84% remaining in continuous remission after 3–4 years [72]. This compares favourably with IFN, where around 30% of patients maintain peripheral blood remission at 4 years [141]. Patients relapsing after an initial response may in some, but not all, cases respond to further DCF [35].

Toxicity Historically, a number of severe toxic effects have been associated with DCF treatment. However, the profound marrow suppression and severe renal or CNS disease that complicated previous regimes are not now seen [41].

Nonetheless, deaths during DCF therapy are reported in most trials. The principal cause of this mortality is neutropenia-related infection. There are two main causes of such neutropenia. Firstly, suppression of both granulocytes and lymphocytes may be a direct result of DCF treatment (significant neutropenia develops in 45% of patients

[41]). Secondly, the disease itself may cause neutropenia. In the past, many patients treated with DCF had IFN-resistant disease and had experienced especially prolonged and severe neutropenias. Thus, it is difficult to separate treatment-related deaths from those related to the disease itself. It is clear, however, that infective symptoms occur in up to 30% of DCF-treated patients and that in 9–15% these are severe [41]. In contrast, the widely recognised persistent lymphopenia induced by DCF is not apparently related to increased infection [376].

Among other side effects, nausea and vomiting are the most frequently reported symptoms, and these may require prophylactic anti-emetics [72]. A skin rash occurs in up to 70% of patients. In most cases, however, such symptoms are not severe and rarely require treatment withdrawal.

6.4.2
Therapeutic activity of CDA

Practical considerations

Treatment regime: 0.1 mg/kg administered daily by continuous infusion for 7 days.

Mortality: similar to DCF; neutropenia-related deaths reported.

Side effects: major/common effects are neutropenia and culture-negative fever; minor or uncommon reported effects include phlebitis, epidermal necrolysis, neuropathy, confusion, weakness, myalgia and cardiac effects.

Response: clearance of HCs from peripheral blood is seen within days; median time to peripheral blood remission is around 10–15 weeks, with maximal effect in 6 months.

Follow up: marrow biopsy to define response, but results not clearly predictive of relapse.

Background Although CDA has been introduced more recently than DCF, it has been used in the treatment of HCL since 1987, and there is now considerable experience with its administration, effectiveness and toxicity. Unfortunately, no direct comparative trials with other agents have been reported.

Administration A single course of CDA, administered for seven consecutive days at a dose of 0.1 mg/kg by continuous IV infusion is highly effective [293]. Alternative routes of administration, such as oral and subcutaneous, are possible [62, 197].

Remission induction In the largest ongoing study, 144 patients have been treated with CDA; 85% have achieved CR and 12% PR, while 2% have failed to respond [294]. Response rates are fairly rapid, but maximal effects may not be seen until six months after initial treatment [102]. Other studies have found similar results, and the combined findings of six trials indicate an overall response rate of 94% (CR 82%, PR 12%, no response 5%) [318]. Achievement of remission appears to be independent of prior treatment with either splenectomy or αIFN [294]. However, no data have been presented for subjects showing primary resistance to IFN. Between 20 and 50% of patients in apparent CR by conventional staining can be shown to have HCs in the marrow by more sensitive techniques [95, 100, 109, 154,

353]. Furthermore, a substantial number of patients in apparent CR have minor unexplained splenic enlargement detected on imaging [353]. Patients with residual marrow disease may be at increased risk of relapse [353].

Length of remission Remission after CDA appears well maintained. Reported relapse rates vary between series [227, 294], and it is too early to make clear comparisons with other treatments. However, present data indicate that relapse rates are lower than those seen after αIFN treatment, and are likely to be comparable or superior to those following DCF. A second course of CDA may be effective in reinducing CR or PR in relapsed patients [227].

Toxicity Dose-related marrow suppression is the most serious toxicity associated with CDA. At present dose regimes, neutropenia occurs after around a week of treatment, with a mean nadir of $0.4 \times 10^9/l$ [294]. Although red cells and platelets are also suppressed, transfusion support is rarely required. The extent of neutropenia relates to the degree of marrow suppression present before commencing therapy [318]. CDA, like DCF, causes a prolonged CD4 lymphopenia. In HCL this does not appear to be of clinical significance [199, 227, 327], although a high incidence of opportunistic infection has been reported when other disorders have been treated [27].

Fever occurs in up to half of CDA patients; in the majority, it is of short duration, occurring after around six days of treatment. This short-term, culture-negative fever is most common in individuals with a large tumour bulk. This fever has been attributed to cytokine release during lysis of HCs, but this remains unproven [294]. Infections occur in 10–39% of patients, and fatal outcomes have been reported. Serious or fatal infection is frequently opportunistic in nature [42, 102, 197], and may reflect the prior immune suppression associated with the disease. Fatal bacteraemia may also occur [42]. A significant proportion of patients require hospital admission after CDA [294].

6.4.3
Fludarabine

Fludarabine has become widely used in the treatment of CLL and related disorders. Experience of its use in HCL is very limited, but a number of reports indicate that the agent has significant activity in the disease [202, 220]. However, such studies have involved relatively few patients, who have often been resistant to other treatment modalities. It is difficult, therefore, to compare the activity of fludarabine with that of the other purine analogues in HCL.

It is clear, however, that at the doses employed in CLL the side effects of fludarabine are relatively marked. Fever occurs in 59%, while 35% show definite infection; there is a 36% incidence of nausea and vomiting [312]. In terms of toxicity, therefore, present dose schedules provide no advantage over DCF or CDA.

Fludarabine should, however, be regarded as an effective drug in the treatment of HCL, and may be useful in cases resistant to other drugs, or when alternative forms of treatment are unsuitable.

6.4.4
Choice of purine analogue drug in HCL

Although fludarabine may prove to be very effective, experience with its use in HCL is very limited. The principal choice at present, therefore, is between DCF and CDA. The overall response rates to DCF and CDA are around 90%, with low rates of early relapse. CDA may show a slightly higher response rate, but trials have not been comparative and differences appear small. For both drugs remission appears well maintained with low relapse rates, at least in the short term. In this regard, there is more experience with DCF, and several series report that most patients remain in remission beyond 4 years. Following relapse, a proportion of patients respond to re-treatment with the same agent. It has been reported that patients primarily or secondarily resistant to DCF may respond to CDA, but such responses are not always seen.

CDA has a simpler administration regime and can include subcutaneous or oral routes. In terms of toxicity, the most serious effect of both drugs is neutropenia and subsequent infection. The principal factor determining neutropenia appears to be the degree of marrow suppression present before therapy; it is difficult, therefore, to determine whether or not either agent offers any advantage in this regard. CDA has a lower incidence of other side effects, but culture-negative fever is common and may necessitate hospital admission.

Until the drugs are compared directly, apparent differences in efficacy must be considered unproven. However, perhaps the best guide to the likely future position of DCF and CDA is the perception of clinicians. A questionnaire of community based oncologists in New York, New Jersey and Connecticut revealed that 78% considered CDA to be the primary choice of non-emergency therapy in HCL [15]. In other geographical areas, preferences may differ according to availability, experience and cost. However, the preferences expressed in the New York, New Jersey and Connecticut study illustrate the strong case that has been made in favour of CDA.

6.5
The use of colony-stimulating factors in HCL

Summary

- G-CSF is effective both in restoring counts and resolving infection; GM-CSF has been less well studied, but limited studies suggest a similar efficacy.
- G-CSF effectively supports counts in neutropenic patients treated with IFN. There are no current data on the use of G-CSF during treatment with purine analogue drugs, but GM-CSF provides no benefit during CDA therapy.
- HCs express receptors for GM-CSF and M-CSF. Although there is no evidence that either cytokine promotes the proliferation or survival of the malignant cell, possible direct effects on the HC should be considered if therapy with either cytokine is planned.

Role of colony-stimulating factors in the cytopenias of HCL In vitro studies have consistently reported impaired myeloid and erythroid colony growth in the presence of HCs or HC-conditioned media. The major element in this impaired growth *in vitro* is the secretion of one or more inhibitory factors by the HC, principally TNFα [112, 238, 355]. In vivo, additional elements such as bone marrow invasion and fibrosis may inhibit normal cell production. However, there is a limited body of evidence pointing to an additional impairment of normal colony-stimulating factor function. In one *in vitro* study it has been shown that, although removal of TNFα partially restores normal colony growth in HCL, full restoration requires the addition of GM-CSF [121]. Furthermore, levels of M-CSF are not raised despite the presence of profound monocytopenia in the disease, perhaps indicating an impairment of the normal feedback loop for the cytokine [194].

Use of colony-stimulating factors in the therapy of HCL G-CSF is highly effective in correcting the neutropenia of HCL. Doses ranging from 2 µg/kg to 7 µg/kg have been reported to induce normal numbers of circulating neutrophils [132, 134, 243], with resolution of infections when present [132, 243]. A rare treatment failure has been reported in the presence of very severe neutropenia [243], and in one case treatment had to be discontinued after Sweet's syndrome developed [132]. However, the neutrophil count rapidly falls when G-CSF is discontinued [243]; thus the cytokine can only be recommended for short-term administration.

There are therefore two important instances where G-CSF may be of benefit. The first is in the treatment of acute infection. The second is as an adjunct to support neutrophil counts during initial therapy in HCL. In this latter regard, G-CSF has been

Table 6.2 Summary of treatment response of HCL to the major forms of therapy

	Treatment employed*			
	Splenectomy	Interferon	DCF	CDA
Peripheral blood remission	40–60%	~80%	>85%	>90%
Bone marrow remission	Rare	10%**	75–80%[+]	~85%[+]
Median time to treatment failure[†]	18 months	30 months	>75% remain in remission after 3–4 years	Not evaluable; probably similar to DCF
Percentage achieving sustained remission[‡]	10	20	High, percentage not yet evaluable	High, percentage not yet evaluable
Principal side effects	Surgical risk, infection	Initial 'flu', fatigue	Neutropenia, nausea and vomiting	Neutropenia, fever

*Note that the results given for each form of therapy do not represent direct comparative trials. Trials may employ different patient populations, while assessment of remission and evaluation of failure may also differ between studies. The figures given are average levels from various trials. For a more detailed description refer to the text.
**Marrow remission in IFN-treated subjects varies widely between studies. Residual HCs are found in most cases on close examination, but the significance of such cells is unclear.
[+]Minimal residual disease is present in a significant proportion of cases.
[†]Treatment failure represents time to HCL-related death or to institution of second therapy. Reappearance of HCs or clinical deterioration may occur significantly earlier.
[‡]Sustained remission refers to stable disease, either in partial or in complete clinical remission.

successfully used to restore counts before IFN therapy, and then support neutrophil levels during continuing IFN therapy [134]. Whether G-CSF is effective in combination with DCF or CDA has not as yet been reported.

GM-CSF has been less well studied, although in a single case neutrophil counts were restored [239]. GM-CSF does not support counts or reduce neutropenic fever during CDA treatment. There have been no reports of the administration of M-CSF to HCL patients.

Direct effects of colony-stimulating factors on HCs CSFs are multifunctional molecules and, in addition to colony-stimulating activity, exert a wide range of effects on mature cell types. Furthermore, it is becoming recognised that receptors for these cytokines may be expressed on non-myeloid lineages and on malignant cells [405]. In this regard, we have shown that HCs express the receptor for M-CSF

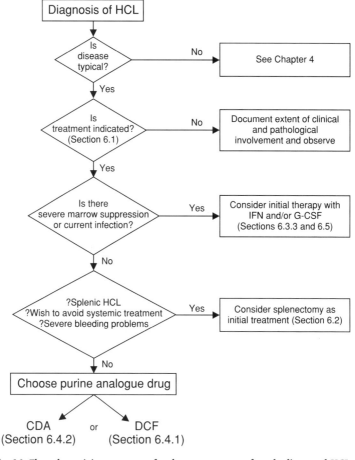

Fig. 6.1. Flow chart giving a strategy for the management of newly diagnosed HCL.

[362] and that the cytokine induces HC motility [49]. We have also detected receptors for GM-CSF on the surface of HCs [364].

The direct effects of these CSFs on HCs *in vitro* are discussed in Section 7.7.5. Whether GM-CSF or M-CSF might have beneficial or adverse effects on HCs *in vivo* has not been determined. However, the possibility of direct effects of CSFs on HCs should be considered if the clinical use of these agents is planned.

6.6
Overview of therapeutic options

Summary of major treatment choices Table 6.2 and Fig. 6.1 summarize the treatment options for HCL.

6.7
Treatment after failure of primary treatment option

Although prolonged remissions are usually seen after treatment with purine analogue drugs, a proportion of patients are primarily resistant to these agents and it is probable that a significant proportion of those entering remission will ultimately relapse. At the time of writing, it is not possible to give clear guidance on how to treat such patients, but Table 6.3 gives details of strategies that may be helpful.

6.8
Other treatment options

A wide range of treatments have been employed in HCL. All are considerably less effective than current treatments and are thus largely of historical interest. Such treatments are summarised in Table 6.4.

Table 6.3 Treatment after failure of preferred option

Failed primary treatment	Options after failure
Splenectomy	All other options effective.
IFN	Primary resistance or acquired non-immune resistance: splenectomy or purine analogue. Immune-mediated resistance: alternative form of IFN or purine analogue. Relapse: Reinduction with IFN or purine analogue.
DCF	Primary resistance: CDA effective in some cases; no data for IFN or splenectomy. Relapse: reinduction with DCF or CDA may be effective.
CDA	Primary resistance: a second treatment with CDA may be effective; fludarabine reported to be successful in one case. Relapse: reinduction with CDA may be effective. No data for use of IFN, DCF or splenectomy.

Table 6.4 'Historical' treatments'

Treatment	Reference	Comment
Cytotoxic therapy:		Sensitivity varies, good cytotoxic effect may be seen but prolonged cytopenias and poor recovery of neutrophils are usual.
examples:		
Chlorambucil	[137]	2/4 mg alternative days for 6 months. Improvement seen, mainly in Hb and platelets; neutropenia and risk of infection are unchanged.
Cyclophosphamide	[67]	Dose not given. Results reported to be similar to chlorambucil.
Combination chemo or anthracycline	[89]	Variable response, prolonged cytopenia and poor response of neutrophils.
Lithium	[32, 231]	One case report of complete response; further reports of neutropenia improving.
Leukapheresis	[106, 399]	Post-splenectomy patients, $n = 4$ total. Total of 10+ cycles in high-count and low-count subjects. Haematological improvement maintained >1 year; infective complications improved.
Anti-TNFα	[177]	Modest reduction in tumour burden; poorly tolerated ($n = 3$).
Bone marrow transplant	[78]	Apparent cure, but single case with identical twin donor ($n = 1$).

CHAPTER 7

The Hairy Cell

Summary: Cytology and cytochemistry

- The diagnosis of HCL rests on the identification of HCs; a combination of characteristics – typical nuclear, membrane and cytoplasmic features – should be sought.
- The membrane hairs are the most obvious feature and are distinguished from those in other conditions by their frequency and fine nature. However, hairs may be absent from some or occasionally most HCs.
- The principal cytochemical feature of HCs is TRAP, and 95% of cases show strong positivity in some or all HCs. Weak TRAP reactivity may occur in related conditions.

7.1
Cytology

Hairy cells derive their name from the irregular fine cytoplasmic projections that extend for variable distances from the periphery. It is, however, a combination of characteristics that identifies the HC in Romanowsky preparations. The eccentric nucleus with its fine chromatin condensation, the pale slate-blue cytoplasm and the fine surface projections all form part of the initial diagnostic impression (Plate 6).

The mononuclear HC is larger than most lymphocytes, with a diameter of 15–30 μm and a modal cell volume by electronic measurement of approximately 450 μm³ [39]. In Romanowsky preparations the surface projections often produce no more than an ill-defined fringe to the cell outline: it is the frequency and fine nature of the hairs that distinguish them from the surface projections often seen on a variety of other cell types [336]. However, in some patients surface hairs may be completely absent from a proportion, or even the majority, of recognisably pathological cells (Fig. 7.1); these cells can be identified by their nuclear structure and cytoplasmic staining.

The nuclear–cytoplasmic ratio is generally intermediate between the high ratio of lymphocytes and the low ratio of monocytes, macrophages and some leukaemic monocyte precursors. The eccentrically placed nucleus is usually round or oval; there may be indentation or cleavage, and a folded or kidney shape may be seen. The nuclear chromatin is finely dispersed and nucleoli are not conspicuous.

The cytoplasm stains a slate-blue with Romanowsky stains, a colour intermediate between the sky-blue of the lymphocyte cytoplasm and the grey of the monocyte, and less basophilic than the cytoplasm of most immature haemic cells. The structure sometimes appears homogeneous, but patchy variations in density are common and

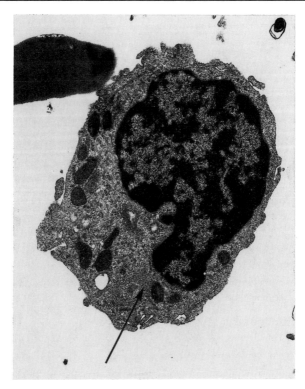

Fig. 7.1. A 'bald' hairy cell. The presence of a ribosome – lamellar complex (arrow) identifies the cell as an HC.

vacuoles are frequently seen [73]. The cytoplasm may occasionally contain small azurophilic granules [73].

7.2
Cytochemistry

7.2.1
Tartrate-resistant acid phosphatase (TRAP)

Seven isoenzymes of acid phosphatase are demonstrable in normal and pathological leukocytes by gel electrophoresis [234]. Isoenzyme 5, although not completely specific for HCL, is present in large amounts in HCs and constitutes the major isoenzyme type [185, 204]. The subcellular location of the enzyme and its potential biological functions are discussed in Section 7.6.3. Isoenzyme 5 is resistant to inactivation by L(+) tartrate and so can be demonstrated by a simple cytochemical method.

TRAP cytochemistry on blood/marrow smears If performed carefully, TRAP staining can be of great value diagnostically (Plate 7). However, consistent cytochemical demonstration of TRAP activity in HCs requires attention to several technical

Table 7.1 TRAP reactivity in relevant haematological and non-haematological cell types

Other strongly positive cell types	Gaucher cells, osteoclastoma
Normal leukocytes (weak reactivity)	Activated B cells, mantle zone cells, granuloma macrophages
Malignant haematological cells (occasional strong reaction)	Histiocytic disorders, Waldenström's macro-globulinaemia
Malignant haematological cells (weak reactivity)	B-CLL, B-PLL, T-PLL, T-ALL, ATLL
Relevant non-reactive cells	Monocytes (blood and marrow), macrophages in liver, spleen and node

Source: [99].

factors. These have been carefully reviewed by Janckila et al. [183] and are presented in Appendix A.

TRAP detection on paraffin sections Cytochemical detection of TRAP is not possible on formalin-fixed paraffin-embedded tissue sections since enzyme activity is destroyed by the fixation process [187]. Recently, however, successful immunohistochemical localisation of TRAP has been reported using an antibody that recognises the denatured form of the enzyme [187].

Interpretation of TRAP The interpretation of TRAP cytochemistry requires attention to a number of important points. Most leukocytes contain tartrate-sensitive acid phosphatases. It is therefore necessary to show that these have been successfully inhibited in any TRAP preparation. This is readily done by showing reactive HCs together with negative adjacent neutrophils. In typical HCL, at least 95% of cases are positive for TRAP. However, within a given case, positivity can vary between 5 and 95% of cells, and the intensity of reaction between cells may also vary considerably (reviewed in [99]). Moderate TRAP reactivity may also be seen in other leukaemic cells and in certain normal leukocyte types. The reactivity of TRAP in such cells rarely causes diagnostic difficulty, but it is important to be aware of such potential reactivity. The relevant reactive and non-reactive cell types are outlined in Table 7.1.

Strong TRAP positivity remains highly suggestive of HCs, and even in cases in which few morphological HCs are present in the peripheral blood, occasional TRAP-positive cells can generally be found.

7.2.2
Other cytochemical techniques

Although a range of cytochemical reactivities of varying specificities have been described, only TRAP is routinely employed in the diagnosis of HCL. The major cytochemical techniques employed in the past and their reactivities are summarised in Table 7.2 (for detailed review see [73]).

Table 7.2 Cytochemical reactivity of HCs using various techniques

Cytochemical technique	Reactivity	Comment
Acid phosphatase	+++/+	Tartrate resistant (see text for use)
Non-specific esterase	++	Granular (fine and coarse)
PAS	++/+	Diffuse or rarely granular
Alkaline phosphatase	0	
Peroxidase	0	May be reactive in unfixed cells
Lysozyme	0	

7.3
Cytogenetics

Summary

- Clonal karyotypic abnormalities occur in around a third of cases, but random changes are also common.
- No single abnormality is characteristic of HCL, but changes involving chromosome 5 are most frequent. A wide range of other karyotypic alterations is reported.
- The significance of cytogenetic abnormalities in HCL is unclear

7.3.1
Frequency of karyotypic abnormalities

Spontaneous metaphases are rare in cultured HCs [198]. However, increasing knowledge of B cell mitogens – and more recently the use of FISH [233] or CD40 proliferation systems [212] – has enabled a more complete knowledge of HCL karyotypes. In a review of all published studies until 1993, karyotypic abnormalities were found in 59 of 141 evaluable cases [198]. This figure includes the results of early studies where few abnormalities were detected. The true incidence remains unclear since recent large studies employing a variety of methodologies have differed quite significantly in the number of abnormalities identified. One study employing B-cell mitogens found a karyotypic abnormality in 67% [153], while a study using a CD40 proliferation system found chromosomal abnormalities in only 19% [212].

7.3.2
Specificity of chromosomal changes

Several chromosomal abnormalities seen in HCL are common to lymphoproliferative disorders in general. These include structural abnormalities with the 14q+ marker involving the heavy-chain locus, structural and numerical abnormalities of chromosome 12, and structural abnormalities involving 11q and 6q [156, 198].

Abnormalities found in HCL but rarely seen in other lymphoproliferative disorders have also been described. The most consistent 'HC-specific' findings involve chromosome 5, the most common being trisomy 5 or structural abnormalities involving 5q13. Such changes were found in 43% of patients in one report [153]. Abnormalities have also been reported which involve chromosomes 1, 2, 7, 19 and 20, but these are less consistently seen [153].

In addition, studies have drawn attention to the existence of multiple abnormalities of karyotype within a given case of HCL. Random chromosomal deletions are common and non-clonal cytogenetic changes are frequently seen [153, 212]. Multiple clones with unrelated or partially related abnormalities are frequently identified in cells from a single patient.

7.3.3
Possible significance of karyotypic changes in HCL

The highly consistent clinical behaviour of HCL suggests a specific genetic abnormality. However, cytogenetic studies have not so far identified such a lesion.

Of those chromosomal changes shared with other lymphoproliferative disorders, the 14q+ marker has been best characterised. In mantle zone lymphoma and in cases of PLL and SLVL, 14q+ forms part of a specific t(11;14) translocation and activates BCL-1 [40]. However, in HCL the donor chromosome for 14q+ appears to be random [40]. Of the more specific findings, the occurrence of multiple karyotypic abnormalities in individual cases and the frequent abnormalities involving chromosome 5 have been the subject of some interest. The multiple, non-related, clonal abnormalities within a given case of HCL do not represent clonal evolution, suggesting instead chromosomal instability [153]. It has been suggested that the abnormalities of chromosome 5 may result in the activation of *ras* p21 or of the dihydrofolate reductase gene, and that these may underlie the chromosomal instability [153].

As for most other mature B cell malignancies, it must at present be concluded that the tumorigenic and prognostic significance of cytogenetic abnormalities in HCL is not clear.

7.4
Ultrastructure

Summary

- The ultrastructural features of the HC are those of a metabolically active cell with frequent vacuoles, vesicles and mitochondria.
- R–L complexes occur in 50% of cases but are not confined to HCL; their function is not known.
- Scanning electron microscopy reveals the unique surface topography of HCs, with a mixture of ruffles, ridges and microvilli.

7.4.1
Transmission electron microscopy

At the ultrastructural level, as at the level of the light microscope, HCs display a characteristic and distinctive appearance (Fig. 7.2) (reviewed in [73]). The fine structural features are those of a metabolically active cell deriving much of its energy from oxidative mitochondrial metabolism.

Fig. 7.2. Hairy cell. Fine microvilli and more broadly-based surface projections are present. The inset shows how in favourable sections, microfibrils are seen entering the microvilli. Vacuoles and vesicles of varying size are particularly prominent in this cell. A centriole (c) is present in transverse section and microtubules are seen converging on the nearby pericentriolar satellites. The eccentric nuclear profile with its peripheral chromatin condensation is typical; a single nucleolus is present.

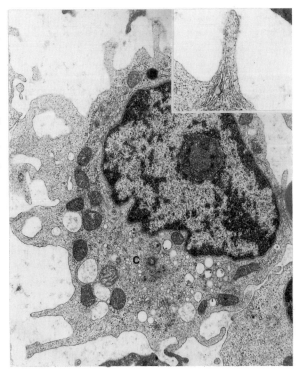

Nucleus In most planes of section, a single nuclear profile with one or more indentations is seen. Peripheral chromatin condensation is slight to moderate, and nucleoli are infrequent. When nucleoli are present they are nearly always single and are not highly developed.

Cytoplasm The surface projections of HCs are a consistent feature and are not critically dependent on optimal fixation, being well seen even after harsh handling methods.

The surface projections are of two main types: numerous fine microvilli and less frequent broadly based structures. In favourable sections, large numbers of microfilaments can be seen entering the microvilli. In most cases, occasional other-wise typical HCs are seen to lack surface projections, and in a few patients such cells are prominent, even when great care is taken with fixation.

The cytoplasm frequently contains numerous vacuoles and vesicles of variable size and shape. In addition, a number of membrane-bound granular structures of varying size and shape may be seen. The most frequent granule type is small and displays an electron-dense core surrounded by a peripheral pale zone. At least some of these granules can be shown to possess acid phosphatase activity and therefore to be lysosomes.

In suitably stained material, the HC can frequently be seen to contain significant amounts of glycogen, which is either scattered diffusely through the cytoplasm as single granules or is sometimes arranged as small collections of particles; this distribution of glycogen accounts for the diffuse and the fine granular PAS positivity of HCs.

HCs contain abundant mitochondria together with modest numbers of ribosomes. A few short strands of rough endoplasmic reticulum (RER) are typically present, and these are frequently associated with any R–L complexes present (see below).

The Golgi apparatus is only moderately developed, consisting of some 3–5 cisternae and a variable number of associated vesicles and vacuoles. Prominent centrioles are frequently seen in the Golgi area, and microtubules, which extend throughout the cytoplasm of HCs, can often be observed converging on the conspicuous pericentriolar satellites. Randomly orientated fibrils are also frequently prominent, especially in the perinuclear area of the cytoplasm.

Ribosome–lamellar complexes These distinctive structures were first described in HCs by Katayama *et al.* [204]. Although R–L complexes may occasionally be observed in a variety of other haematological and non-haematological cell types, they are more common in HCL than in other haematological malignancies [206] and are therefore of diagnostic significance. The function of R–L complexes is unknown, but they are not involved in Ig synthesis since they are unreactive in cells stained immunocytochemically for Ig.

R–L complexes have been reported to occur in approximately 50% of cases of HCL [206] and in from 0.2% to almost 100% of the cells of a given case [206]. As their name suggests, R–L complexes are composed of ribosomal granules associated with an elaborate system of fibrils (the lamellar component) (Figs 7.3, 7.4 and 7.5).

The granules of the complex are identical with the ribosomes in the neighbouring cytoplasm and their RNA content has been demonstrated by a number of studies

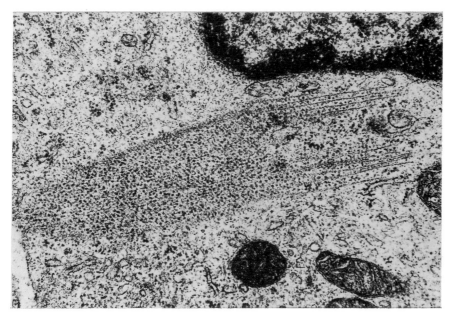

Fig. 7.3. Ribosome–lamellar complex. Longitudinal/transverse section (×37 500). Careful examination reveals a net-like structure.

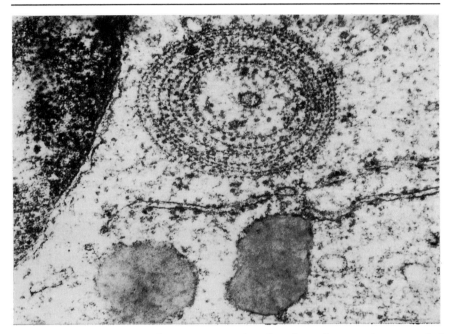

Fig. 7.4. Ribosome–lamellar complex. Transverse section. The coils can be seen to be composed of distinct subunits; ribosomes are concentrically arranged approximately midway between the coils.

(e.g. [10]). In longitudinal section, the lamellar component is seen as multiple (up to eight) parallel straight fibrils arranged on each side of a central core. These fibrils are usually regularly spaced and can sometimes be seen to be continuous with the less regularly arranged fibrils that extend throughout the cytoplasm of HCs [339]. The spaces between fibrils are occupied by parallel rows of ribosomes. In transverse section, the central core is slightly oval in outline and the lamellar component appears as a two-dimensional coiled structure, while the ribosomes are arranged concentrically between the coils [88].

The precise three-dimensional structure giving rise to these appearances is not known, but the R–L complex may represent a cylindrical coiled structure [88] where the coil is composed of a two-dimensional net of fibrils from which ribosomes are suspended [73].

Fibrillary inclusions HCs frequently contain prominent bundles of fibrils. Such fibrils are rare in CLL and their presence in HCL may reflect the cytoskeletal activation now known to be a feature of HCL (Section 7.6.2).

Ultrastructural cytochemistry Some of the acid phosphatase in HCs is not tartrate resistant [185]. This activity is located in lysosomes and has been used to show that HCs can form phagocytic vacuoles around internalised latex particles, and therefore that at least some of the particles are truly phagocytosed.

HCs possess an endogenous peroxidase distinct from myeloperoxidase and catalase. The enzyme is found in the endoplasmic reticulum and the perinuclear cistern, but not in the Golgi apparatus. The peroxidase resembles that demonstrable in the megakaryocytic series, but its function and significance in HCs are unclear.

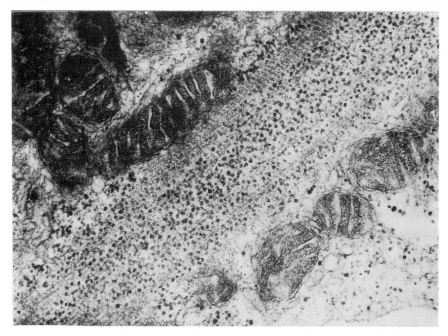

Fig. 7.5. Ribosome–lamellar complex. Oblique section. The net-like structure of the lamellar component is clearly seen at the end of each complex.

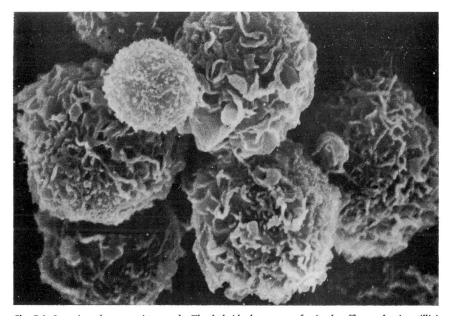

Fig. 7.6. Scanning electron micrograph. The hybrid phenotype of mixed ruffles and microvilli is clearly demonstrated.

7.4.2
Scanning electron microscopy

The surface of HCs is made up of a mixture of ruffles, ridge-like projections and narrow, finger-like microvilli (Fig. 7.6). The surface ruffles resemble those associated with monocytes, while the microvillous projections are like those typical of B-CLL. The surface topography of HCs is therefore distinctive, but its significance is still not clear. It is likely that the complex surface appearances reflect the intrinsic cyto-skeletal activation so characteristic of HCL (see Section 7.6.2).

7.5
Nature of the malignant cell

Summary

- The HC is a mature B cell with an activated phenotype.
- Both light and heavy Ig gene loci are rearranged, with evidence of partial, but atypical, class-switching; somatic mutation has not occurred.
- HCs possess distinctive activation features that are different from those of other activated B-cell types.
- The features of the HC may be regarded as those of a cell that has received a partial but incomplete activation signal, but has been unable to undergo terminal differentiation.

The origin of the malignant hairy cell has been a major source of interest since HCL was first described. The original name 'leukaemic reticuloendotheliosis' reflected the reticuloendothelial distribution and unusual characteristics of the malignant cell. This distribution, together with the phagocytic abilities and peculiar cytoskeletal organisation of the HC, was initially presented as evidence of possible monocytic lineage.

It is now accepted, however, that the HC is a mature B lymphocyte with phenotypic features suggesting cell activation. Nonetheless, a true counterpart of the HC among normal B lymphocytes has not been convincingly demonstrated; and neither the precise stage of differentiation of the HC, nor the origin and nature of its ongoing activated state, has been clearly established. Present knowledge in relation to these factors is reviewed below.

7.5.1
Developmental stage: evidence from immunoglobulin studies

The HC is a mature, activated B cell at a pre-plasma cell stage of differentiation The demonstration that HCs have successfully rearranged the gene loci for both light and heavy chains of Ig [217] defines the HC as a mature B lymphocyte. This ontological position is confirmed by the strong expression by HCs of surface immunoglobulin (sIg). HC sIg shows an approximately equal distribution of κ and λ light chains, suggesting successful maturation at the light-chain loci [48, 191, 211], although unusual rearrangements of light-chain genes have been described [273]. At the heavy-chain locus, class switching has occurred. Ig heavy chains of all classes except IgE have been described on HCs [48, 191, 211]. However, there is an unusual predominance of the IgG3 subtype [211]. Furthermore, unlike other B-lymphocytic cells, HCs may simultaneously express multiple different heavy-chain isotypes, e.g. co-expression of IgD, IgA and IgG [48, 191, 211]. In this context, aberrant rearrangements at the heavy-chain loci have been described [209], but similar changes were also found in CLL and PLL, and their significance is therefore unclear.

HCs do not, however, appear to have differentiated beyond the stage of class switching. There is no evidence that the cells have undergone affinity maturation, since somatic mutation in Ig variable region loci has not been found [388]. Unlike plasma cells, HCs do not secrete large amounts of Ig. However, like CLL cells, HCs possess cytoplasmic Ig (cIg) [48] (Fig. 7.7). Furthermore, on culture, low levels of Ig with an excess of light chains are secreted [143]. Low levels of monoclonal Ig can be found in up to 11% of HCL *in vivo*, but this often does not correlate with the isotype(s) expressed on the surface of the HCs in the individual cases and may not be HC-derived [159, 287].

Such studies strongly suggest that in terms of malignant cell ontogeny the HC has differentiated beyond the level seen in CLL and PLL, where class switching has not occurred. However, the absence of somatic mutation and lack of formation of Ig for secretion place the HC at an earlier stage than that of the myeloma cell. The position of the HC in relation to normal B-cell ontogeny is, however, less straightforward. The possible developmental paths are discussed below.

Is the HC developmental stage compatible with that of a cell that has received a T-dependent antigen signal? Certain characteristics of the HC might suggest that it is at the developmental stage of a mature B lymphocyte that has been activated by exposure to protein antigen with appropriate T-cell help. The cell has progressed to

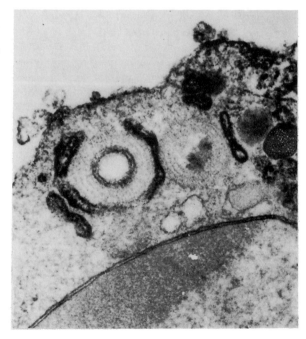

Fig. 7.7. Immunoperoxidase staining with anti-immunoglobulin. Ig is clearly stained within the endoplasmic reticulum, but not in the adjacent ribosome-lamellar complex. The poor preservation is a result of the acetone fixation used to permeabilise the cell.

the developmental stage of Ig heavy-chain class switching, but not to the later stages characterised by somatic mutation or Ig secretion. There are, however, certain problems with such a model.

Firstly, the simultaneous expression of multiple heavy-chain isotypes by a single case of HCL is not compatible with the currently accepted deletion model of Ig class switching. For example, by accepted class switch models, an IgA expressing cell would have deleted DNA coding regions for IgD, IgM and IgG [334]. Thus the co-expression of IgD, IgA and IgG by HCs given as an example above could not have occurred by accepted Ig class-switching mechanisms. Secondly, the particular anatomical location of the HC is not that which would be expected for a cell that has undergone protein antigen stimulation. T-dependent B-cell activation occurs in the T-cell zones of lymphoid tissue. Subsequently, such cells migrate into lymphoid follicles, where cells that successfully complete Ig class switching remain and undergo somatic mutation. Cells that leave the follicle prior to this stage become short-lived plasma cells, which secrete principally IgM and localise to the medullary cords of lymph nodes [248, 245]. Thus, the preferred locations of the HC, particularly splenic red pulp and bone marrow, are not normally occupied by cells derived from T-dependent immune responses. Finally, the IgG3 subtype expression by HCs is not typical of a T-dependent immune response. Cells that develop within lymphoid follicles in association with CD40 ligand principally produce Ig of G1 and G2 subtypes [309] rather than the IgG3 typically displayed by HCs [211].

Is the HC developmental stage compatible with that of a cell that has received a T-independent antigen signal? A more convincing case can be made for the HC representing a B cell activated by a 'T-independent' mechanism. B cells activated *in vivo* by T-independent antigens do not develop within lymphoid follicles. Instead, and like HCs, they are frequently found to co-localise with macrophages within the splenic red pulp [245]. Such cells do not encounter the principal class-switch stimulus, CD40 ligand [309], and in the past have not been thought to undergo Ig class switching. However, recent studies using CD40 ligand knock out mice have shown that T-independent antigenic stimuli can induce Ig class switching and produce all classes of Ig except IgE [48, 191, 211]. Interestingly, IgG3, the major HC Ig form, tends to be the predominant IgG subtype in T-independent immune responses [309].T-independent mechanisms of activation are, however, still unable to explain the simultaneous expression of multiple Ig isotypes by the HC, and there is no direct evidence for the involvement of T-independent antigens in HCL ontology.

However, the signal that has stimulated HCs need not be derived from antigen exposure, but could result from the malignant transformation of the cell. A constitutive oncogenic signal mimicking antigen cross-linkage of the B-cell receptor could induce a 'T-independent' activation of the HC. Such an oncogenic signal might contribute to the ongoing activated nature of the HC.

7.5.2
Developmental stage: evidence from immunophenotypic studies

Immunological markers of B-cell differentiation confirm the mature, but not terminally differentiated, B-cell nature of the HC. Thus, mature B-cell markers normally lost during the terminal stages of B-cell development (e.g. CD19, CD20,

CD40 and FMC7) are present on HCs, while early B-cell markers such as CD10 are absent. HCs express the PCA-1 antigen typical of plasma cells [11], but show no other immunophenotypic features of plasmacytoid differentiation. CD22, whose expression parallels that of sIg, and which is an important co-stimulatory molecule for the B-cell receptor, is expressed at high levels [214]. The immunological phenotype also confirms the evidence that the HC has features of an activated cell. Markers normally lost after B-cell activation, such as CD21 and CD24, are expressed only at low levels, while B-cell activation markers CD25 and CD72 are strongly represented [214].

Other studies have consistently underlined the activated nature of the malignant cell. Successful activation of a cell involves the acquisition of new receptors that allow it to receive important signals from its microenvironment. The cytokine receptor and adhesion receptor expression of the HC show features consistent with such activation (Sections 7.7 and 7.8). Further evidence may be derived from the 'HC-restricted' antigens. Several antibodies initially raised against HCs showed relative specificity for HCL. These antibodies have since been studied in further detail and several have been assigned CD numbers (Table 7.3). As can be seen from the table, most of these HC-restricted Mabs are markers of 'activation'.

Nonetheless, the HC cannot be regarded as a 'typical' activated B cell. As is shown in Table 7.3, two of the three most specific HC markers (CD11c and CD103) principally define activation in non-B cell types. Furthermore, not all features normally associated with B-cell activation are present on HCs. For example, the activation antigen CD38 is not expressed [214], and expression of CD23 is variable [126]. In conclusion, therefore, immunophenotypic studies indicate the activated B-cell nature of the malignant HC, but also emphasise that the activation is specific, and not necessarily shared by other activated B-cell types.

7.5.3
Developmental stage: other approaches

A number of other *in vitro* techniques have contributed to an understanding of the malignant cell. The immunophenotypic data suggesting an activated cell phenotype

Table 7.3 'HC-specific' antibodies

Mab	CD number	Function	Main distribution
S-HCL-1 [321]	sCD22	B-cell-receptor co-signalling.	Pan/late B.
S-HCL-2 [214]	CD72	CD5 ligand	Pan B cell; increased with activation.
S-HCL-3 [321]	CD11c	Adhesion (integrin)	Myeloid/monocytoid cells; increased on activation.
HC1 [214]	Unclustered	?	Also recognises some AML, ALL, CLL.
HC2 [300]	Unclustered	? Role in BCGF responsiveness.	Activated lymphocytes and monocytes.
B-Ly7 [263, 265, 381]	CD103	Adhesion (integrin)	Activated T cells, intraepithelial T cells.

are supported by studies that have described the highly activated state of the cortical actin cytoskeleton (reviewed in Section 7.6.2), and by studies that have suggested high levels of intracellular signalling activity (reviewed in Section 7.6.3).

Of particular interest, however, have been those studies that have aimed to induce further activation or differentiation of the malignant cell. Although a range of stimuli have been described that can alter the cytoskeletal organisation or surface antigen expression of the malignant cell (Sections 5.2.4 and 7.6.2), no cytokine or pharmacological agent has been described that can induce terminal B-cell differentiation in the HC (as determined by significantly increased cytoplasmic or secreted Ig, or by changes in antigen expression [20, 378, 382]). The significance of this 'differentiation block' of HCs is unclear, but it clearly separates the HC from related B-cell malignancies and from normal B cells where, following appropriate stimulation, varying degrees of further or terminal differentiation may be induced (e.g. [98, 124, 382]).

7.6
Membrane, cytoskeletal organisation and signalling

Summary

- The typical hairy appearance of the HC relates to a highly active cytoskeletal organisation.
- The most unusual feature is the organisation of the cortical actin cytoskeleton, which is highly active but remains responsive to additional stimuli. Similar cytoskeletal features may be induced in other lymphocytes by activators of protein kinase C (PKC).
- Studies of the major signalling pathways in HCs suggest high levels of ongoing signalling activity, but again these pathways remain responsive to additional stimuli.

7.6.1
Membrane

The unusual membrane appearances that characterise HCs have prompted a number of studies examining whether the lipid component of HC membranes might partly underlie these appearances. Unusual features of cholesterol biosynthesis were identified in these studies [397] and were related to increased levels and activity of HMG-CoA reductase [398]. However, changes in membrane composition are found in all white cells in HCL and in other malignancies [396]. Moreover the activity of HMG-CoA reductase was not shown to be of primary importance in HCL, and it is now largely accepted that the 'hairy' appearance of the malignant cell relates principally to its cytoskeleton.

7.6.2
Cytoskeleton

The striking 'hairy' surface projections that are so typical of HCs are the result of the peculiar cytoskeletal organisation of the malignant cell. Scanning microscopy reveals that the 'hairs' represent a complex series of microvilli and surface ruffles, present in varying proportions (Section 7.4). Time-lapse video microscopy shows that these ruffles are in a constant state of movement and appear to flow across the cell [50]. Various cytoskeletal structures probably contribute to these appearances.

Intermediate filaments and the microtubular system These two groups of structures are ubiquitous and may be regarded as the principal supporting elements of the cell. The distribution of both structures within lymphocytes is similar; they surround the nucleus and extend into major cell surface projections [242]. Both structures may be disassembled or reassembled during cell division and during dynamic processes such as motility [242].

Microtubules are readily identified in HCs. Transmission electron microscopy (TEM) identifies multiple tubules radiating from one or more pericentriolar areas [73]. As in other lymphoid cell types, dissociation of microtubules with drugs such as colchicine induces HC motility. However, no unique role for microtubules has been demonstrated in HCs.

The intermediate filament vimentin is present in HCs. In other cell types vimentin is thought to provide structural strength, and it is rapidly disassembled during cell motility. It has been reported that the vimentin content of HCs is low in comparison with other B-lineage cells [349, 401], a finding that may be compatible with the enhanced motility and spreading of the malignant HC. It is clear, however, that vimentin fibrils form a well-defined structural array in spread HCs. Fibrils surround the nucleus and extend into long processes but, in contrast to actin, do not extend into the fine hairs of the cell [55].

The actin cytoskeleton The actin cytoskeleton and its binding structures are responsible for the formation of membrane projections and are likely to have an important role in HC appearance and behaviour. Much of the actin within HCs is polymerised into filamentous (F-actin) form, which is particularly apparent in their surface villi and projections [55] (see Fig. 7.2). This contrasts with CLL and normal B cells, where F-actin is less prominent and where its distribution is punctate or confined to the centre of the cell [401].

It is increasingly recognised that the actin cytoskeleton is organised in discrete ways to fulfil specialised functions. These different structural 'arrays' are regulated by specific G-protein-dependent signalling pathways [281].

Arguably, the activity of the 'cortical actin' network is the most unusual feature of HCs. The cortical actin network represents sub-membranous actin filaments that link to particular adhesion receptors and to actin-organising proteins such as spectrin [103]. Membrane structures such as veils, ruffles, pleats, filopodia, microvilli and pseudopodia are dependent on the cortical actin network [3, 38, 348]. Furthermore, the typical HC features of pronounced lectin-induced cap formation and the ability to phagocytose [136] (Figs 7.8 and 7.9) are also cortical actin-dependent events. Exposure of HCs to αIFN induces blunting of hairs and a reduction of cell surface ruffles and has been shown to cause a significant redistribution of spectrin, a protein involved in the organisation of cortical actin [103, 251].

It is also clear, that actin associated with adhesion molecules in the form of focal adhesions is highly active and readily reorganised. HCs stimulated with phorbol ester develop cytoplasmic projections rich in adhesion structures known as podosomes. These podosomes have an intense accumulation of F-actin [55]. Furthermore, HCs

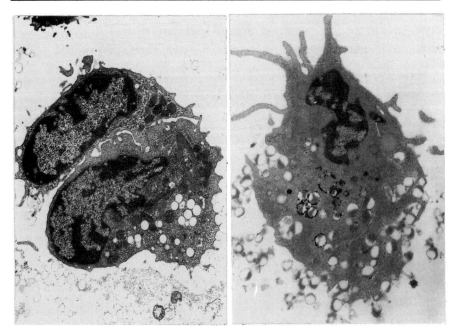

Fig. 7.8. Phagocytosis of latex particles. Left figure: Both HCs contain internalised latex particles. Right figure: Acid phosphatase cytochemistry (lead citrate) identifies the reaction product surrounding the particles, confirming that they are truly phagocytosed.

adherent to different adhesive proteins show very different patterns of actin organisation [50]. This actin distribution parallels the redistribution of integrin adhesion molecules. In motile HCs, F-actin is redistributed along with integrins to the adhesive anterior pole of the cell [49, 50].

Thus, the unusual cytoskeleton of the HC is clearly functional and highly responsive to stimuli. A number of lines of evidence suggest that the unusual and characteristic organisation of the HC cytoskeleton may, in part, reflect the intrinsically 'activated' state of the malignant cell. Normal resting lymphocytes have little ability to spread or migrate. However, following activation, the cells undergo a period of protein synthesis and increase in size; this protein synthesis results in a highly active actin cytoskeleton and enables the cells to spread or migrate [393]. A similar phenomenon occurs following stimulation of normal or malignant lymphocytes with phorbol esters. Such stimulation induces cell spreading and morphological changes in these cells, causing them to resemble HCs [98, 382].

7.6.3
Signalling

Specific intracellular signals are generated through the interaction of a cell with its external environment, or as a result of internal cellular events. Such signals are

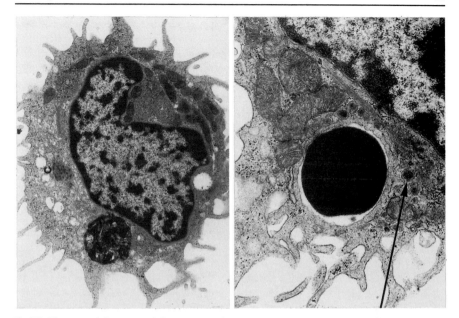

Fig. 7.9. Phagocytosis by HCs. Left figure: HC. A dense membrane-bound structure is present, but the contents are so altered that it is not possible to determine if it is an autophagic or phagocytic vacuole. Right figure: an autophagocytosed erythrocyte is seen. Several granules (e.g. the arrowed structure) are present nearby, and these, in favourable sections, can be seen fusing with the phagocytotic vesicle.

central to the behaviour of both normal and malignant cells. The study of such signals is a rapidly expanding field. Present knowledge of signalling in HCs is incomplete; however, the results of limited studies do provide some insights into HC biology.

Most studies of signalling in HCL have related to PKC. It has been repeatedly shown that CLL cells, NHL cells or normal B cells, when stimulated with PKC activators such as phorbol ester or bryostatin, develop 'hairy-cell-like' features [7, 8, 108, 124, 382]. Such features variably include the development of cytoplasmic processes, expression of TRAP, increased expression of sIg, and the expression of 'HC markers', principally CD11c, CD22, CD25 and B-ly7. It is, however, important to recognise that such cells only partially resemble HCs. Morphologically, the cells only partly resemble HCs, and often display 'non-hairy' features such as expression or retention of CD5 on the cell surface. Moreover, when HCs themselves are stimulated by phorbol ester, different morphological changes occur such as the extension of long dendritic processes; such changes are not seen in other cell types [55].

A second area that has generated some interest has been the study of intracellular free calcium and serine/threonine kinases. Compared with related cell types, the free intracellular calcium level in HCs is elevated. This has been related to high levels of serine/threonine phosphorylation of certain cellular proteins, principally CD20 [127], through the action of the calcium-activated kinase, calcium/calmodulin-dependent kinase II [129].

Finally, attention has been drawn to the activity of the tyrosine protein kinase (TPK)/phosphatase system in HCL. The baseline level of tyrosine phosphorylation in HCL does not differ from that of related B-cell malignancies [221] but, following cell stimulation, the tyrosine phosphorylation pattern of HCs differs markedly from that found in related disorders. Moreover, despite the unremarkable pattern of tyrosine phosphorylation in unstimulated HCs, two reports have emphasised that there are high levels of activity of src and src-related kinases in cell lysates [244, 246]; these findings suggest a high level of activity in the TPK/phosphatase system.

The identity of the tyrosine phosphatases involved in HCL has not been established, but a number of interesting observations have been made. CD45 is a widely expressed surface marker on leukocytes, but is particularly strongly expressed by HCs, showing a characteristic distribution on the hairs of the malignant cell [254]. CD45 is now recognised to possess tyrosine protein phosphatase activity and is well placed to control the activity of membrane-associated TPKs [54]. A second potentially important molecule is TRAP. TRAP expression is acquired by lympho-cytes following activation and is a characteristic feature of HCL (Section 7.2.1). It has recently been reported that TRAP has protein tyrosine phosphatase activity in vitro and in vivo [186]. This raises the possibility that the enzyme has an important role in HCL signalling. However, the fact that most, if not all, TRAP is localised to intracellular vesicles/lysosomes [99] is difficult to reconcile with a major signalling role for the molecule.

Overall, these results confirm that certain of the features that characterise HCs may be attributed to cell activation. However, since phorbol esters activate a wide range of signalling pathways, such stimulation cannot be taken as evidence for a primary role for PKC in the activation or malignant nature of HCL. The capacity of HCs to respond to stimulation with phorbol esters emphasises that the cells are 'incompletely' activated and remain highly responsive to additional signals. Similarly, serine/threonine kinase activity is readily modified in response to external signals. For example, phosphorylation of CD20 is enhanced by low molecular weight (LMW) BCGF and opposed by αIFN [128, 129]. Studies of the function of tyrosine kinases in HCs have been limited, but it has been shown that M-CSF receptor signalling in HCs involves TPK pathways [363] and that such signalling induces pronounced morphological changes in the malignant cell [49].

7.7
Response to cytokines

Summary

- The HC is equipped with a distinctive array of cytokine receptors.
- The principal cytokines and functions described thus far are BCGF (pro-liferation), TNFα (proliferation and survival), M- and GM-CSF (motility and adhesion) and IL-2 (function not clear).

The malignant HC is equipped with a range of receptors for various lymphoid and myeloid growth factors. The roles of some factors in HC biology have been examined in detail; the importance of other factors is only beginning to emerge.

7.7.1
Low molecular weight B-cell growth factor

LMW-BCGF promotes the proliferation of in vitro-activated normal B lymphocytes, and has consistently been shown to promote proliferation of cultured HCs [113, 369]. In vivo, BCGF may be an important growth factor for HCs, either as a paracrine factor secreted by T cells [299] or as an autocrine growth factor secreted by HCs themselves [114]. In addition to these direct proliferative effects, BCGF may also enhance the proliferative response of HCL cells to other growth factors. LMW-BCGF increases secretion of TNFα by HCs, thereby potentially enhancing autocrine TNF-induced proliferation [112]. BCGF also increases expression of the IL-2 receptor α-chain CD25, thereby also potentially enhancing any effect of IL-2 [119].

The mechanism by which BCGF promotes HC proliferation is not clear, although two antigens have been associated with BCGF responses in other cell types. The antigen identified by Mab B8.7 is associated with BCGF-induced proliferation and is consistently detected on HCs [125, 203]. CD23 is also implicated in the BCGF effect, but in HCs is variably expressed and does not seem to be required for BCGF responsiveness [126]. Some details of BCGF signalling have been determined. The cytokine quantitatively and qualitatively alters the expression of the developmentally important B-cell calcium channel CD20. Furthermore, following exposure to LMW-BCGF, CD20 expression is upregulated and is phosphorylated on serine/threonine residues [9, 127]. It is unclear whether such changes are the primary determinant of BCGF-induced HC proliferation. The signalling changes induced by BCGF are opposed by IFN and have been implicated in the therapeutic action of that cytokine (Section 5.2.3).

7.7.2
Tumour Necrosis Factor

HCs synthesise and secrete both TNFα and TNFβ [85, 161]. Little is known concerning TNFβ, but limited studies have not demonstrated any proliferative effects [43]. TNFα, however, has been the subject of considerable interest. Malignant HCs may possess both high and low affinity receptors for TNFα. Thus, only the high affinity TNF receptor is present on ex vivo peripheral blood HCs [369]; following stimulation in vitro, both high and low affinity receptors become expressed [164]. High and low affinity soluble receptors for TNFα occur in HCL plasma [96].

Direct effects of TNFα on HCs Binding of TNFα to its receptor at the HC surface is followed, within 2 hours, by receptor internalisation and mRNA synthesis [28]. Protein synthesis follows within 16 hours. The signalling pathway involves the NFκ B molecule [180]. Early consequences of this biosynthetic activity include proto-oncogene synthesis [168] and, within 48 hours, the expression and translation of mRNA for TNFα itself [83]. TNFα also induces HC proliferation, but detectable proliferation commences only after day 6 [83]. In prolonged culture, the survival of malignant cells is enhanced in the presence of TNFα [319].

The capacity of HCs to synthesise TNFα and the proliferative response induced by the cytokine establish a potential autocrine proliferative cycle in HCL. However, TNF-induced proliferation requires relatively high levels of cytokine. Such levels do not occur in *in vitro* culture, and have not been found in plasma or in bone marrow aspirates. It is possible, however, that levels sufficient to induce proliferation are generated locally within areas of HC infiltration. The delayed proliferative response to TNFα contrasts with the action of the cytokine on other cell types; this implies that the signalling process that generates HC proliferation requires the generation of a secondary signalling element [28], or of secondary cytokine. In this latter respect, a role for intracellular IL-6 has been proposed [21].

Finally, the cytokine enhances survival of HCs [83, 319]. Overall, therefore, the direct effects of TNFα are likely to favour HC growth and accumulation.

Circulating TNF in HCL Circulating levels of TNFα found in HCL blood and bone marrow are much higher than those found in most other haematological malignancies [111, 226]. The major source of this cytokine appears to be direct release by HCs [111]. In addition to the autocrine proliferative activity described above, a further consequence of this circulating TNFα is the suppression of other bone marrow elements.

Suppression of colony forming elements by HCs is widely recognised [184, 355]. Such suppression is almost certainly multi-factorial and involves direct invasion/ fibrosis of bone marrow [184], deficiency of CSFs [121] and secreted inhibitory factors [355]. Evidence from *in vitro* studies would suggest that TNFα is the major, and perhaps the sole, secreted factor responsible for this inhibition (e.g. [112]).

TNFα and therapy of HCL αIFN inhibits the proliferative response of HCs to TNFα [28]. This inhibition may partly underlie the therapeutic action of IFN (discussed in Section 5.2.2). The possibility of direct anti-TNF treatment has also been investigated. Huang *et al.* employed anti-TNFα antibodies in HCL patients [177]. Unfortunately, the immunogenicity of the antibody preparations employed caused significant patient intolerance, and the effects of antibody on circulating TNFα levels proved difficult to interpret. Nonetheless, a modest reduction in spleen size was reported during treatment and cytopenias were reported to improve.

7.7.3
Interleukin-2

The IL-2 receptor in HCL In common with normal activated B cells, HCs express the IL-2 receptor at their cell surface. Typical HCs express the IL-2 receptor α-chain (CD25, TAC) at levels of around 2000 molecules per cell [22]. The α-chain alone binds IL-2 with low affinity, but does not transduce any intracellular signal [356]. The α-chain is also released by HCs into the plasma, where its concentration is up to 60-fold higher than in normal individuals [323].

Formation of functional (signal transducing) IL-2 receptor requires either a dimeric association of β and γ chains (intermediate affinity receptor) or a trimeric association of α, β and γ chains (high affinity receptor) [356]. All three chains have now been identified on HCs [94, 370]. However, β chain expression is considerably lower than α expression, allowing only a limited number (~30/cell) of functional high affinity receptors to be formed [53]. HCs upregulate α-chain expression in response to TNFα [161] or IL-2 itself [94], but present limited data suggest that β chains are not upregulated.

Role of IL-2 The presence of functionally competent IL-2 receptor suggests an important role for the cytokine in HC biology. However, it has proved difficult to ascribe clear functional effects to the cytokine. No consistent effect on surface antigen expression has been found [145]. Although recent data suggest that the cytokine can induce low-level proliferation *in vitro* [370], IL-2 is far less effective in inducing HC proliferation than are TNFα or BCGF. Similarly, IL-2 has no consistent effect on other major areas of HC biology; HC survival is not enhanced [319] and Ig secretion is unchanged [20].

The apparent excess levels of surface or secreted IL-2α chain in HCL are also unexplained. It has been suggested that IL-2 binding by cell-surface or secreted chain serves to reduce levels of circulating IL-2, thereby contributing to the T-cell dysfunction observed in HCL [380]. However, calculations of binding capacity have not supported such a role. In active HCL, only the trimeric form of receptor has sufficient affinity and capacity to reduce circulating concentrations of cytokine [53].

For the present, therefore, no clear role can be assigned to the different IL-2 receptor components. HCL-like cell lines [307] and HCs themselves [308] are protected by IL-2 from NK or cytotoxic T-cell destruction, but the mechanism of such protection is unclear. Finally, recent reports suggest that the β and γ chains of the IL-2 receptor form part of a receptor for an alternative interleukin (IL-15) [17]. How these findings may apply to HCL remains to be determined.

7.7.4
Other Interleukins

Many of the interleukins are important in the controlled differentiation and proliferation of mature B cells, or are proliferative factors for their malignant counterparts. The ontological position of the HC as a 'pre-plasma cell' identifies it as a potential target for a number of these factors. Although IL-2 has been the principal area of interest in HCL, limited studies have examined the role of various other members of the interleukin family in the disorder. No clear functional importance has been identified for any of these factors, but the results of studies undertaken are given in Table 7.4.

Table 7.4 Interleukins potentially involved in HC biology

Interleukin	Role in HCL	references
IL-1 IL-3	Not recognised lymphokines. No identified role in HCL. Serum IL-1β levels raised in HCL in common with other malignancies; significance not known.	[20, 148, 319]
IL-4 IL-5	Recognised lymphokines for mature B cells. No evidence for effect on HC differentiation or survival. IL-4 may have minor direct or indirect effects on proliferation.	[20, 148, 249, 319]
IL-6	HCs express IL-6 receptor and bind the cytokine, and may produce IL-6 after TNFα stimulation. The cytokine does not affect proliferation, differentiation or survival of HCs (c.f. effects on plasma cells).	[20, 148, 319]
IL-10	RNA message for the cytokine is expressed by HCs.	[213]
IL-15	Express receptor. Function unknown.	See Section 7.7.3

7.7.5
Myeloid growth factors

It is now clear that receptors for CSFs may be expressed on various non-myeloid lineages and on malignant cells [405]. HCs express the receptors for at least two of these factors on their surface: M-CSF [363] and GM-CSF [364].

Expression of M-CSF receptor by HCs appears to be related to the activated state of the malignant cell since the receptor is also expressed by low density (activated) tonsillar B cells and on *in vitro*-activated peripheral blood cells [362]. M-CSF does not cause HCs to proliferate or differentiate, but does cause an extensive rearrangement of cellular actin and leads to enhanced cell movement [49] (Fig. 7.10).

In contrast, the presence of the receptor for GM-CSF on HCs appears to be a feature of their differentiation state since the receptor is also expressed on other mature B-cell neoplasms and on normal plasma cells [364]. Like M-CSF, GM-CSF does not affect the proliferation or differentiation of HCs but, in contrast to M-CSF,

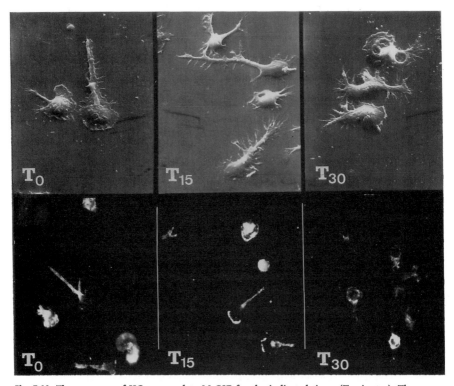

Fig. 7.10. The response of HCs exposed to M-CSF for the indicated times (T minutes). The upper panel shows scanning electron micrographs that illustrate the initial elongation phase (0–15 min) and the later more rounded form (>30 min). The lower panel shows the reorganisation of actin during the same period. Actin is initially localised to the body or tail of the cell, but during elongation rapidly redistributes to the anterior pole before its more diffuse redistribution after 30 min.

the cytokine appears to reduce HC motility, causing a rapid decrease in spreading and adhesion, with a clear reduction in HC motility in *in vitro* assays [364].

The precise role of the CSFs in HC function *in vivo* is unclear, but the two cytokines may have important and contrasting roles in directing the tissue migration of the malignant cell.

7.8
Adhesion and tissue localisation

Summary

- HCs express a wide and distinctive range of adhesion receptors that allow the cell to interact strongly with cell or matrix ligands in the tissue microenvironment.
- The distinctive integrins of HCs have been most widely studied, and they at least partly contribute to the unusual tissue distribution of the malignant cell.

The unique tissue distribution and tissue modification that characterise HCL have been major areas of interest. Recent advances in the understanding of the adhesive behaviour of cells have given some insight into the mechanisms that underlie the migratory behaviour of HCs.

7.8.1
Non-integrin adhesion receptors

An increasingly wide range of cell surface adhesion receptors are now recognised to control the adhesive behaviour of cells. Most belong to the integrin, selectin or Ig superfamilies, but a range of other receptors are also known. HCs express adhesion receptors from each of the major groups at their surface.

Ig superfamily adhesion molecules mediate highly specific interactions and are frequently involved in immune recognition [337]. Important members of the Ig superfamily such as MHC class II, ICAM-1 and CD22 are variably expressed by HCs [214]. Although the specific function of these molecules in HC biology has been little investigated, their presence emphasises the capacity of HCs to interact with a wide range of other haemopoietic cell types. A fourth member – the receptor for aggregated IgG (FCγRII/CD 32) – is consistently and strongly expressed in a highly avid form (Fig. 7.11). The specific biological relevance of this expression is not clear. However, the finding has been of importance in two regards. Firstly, the ability to bind aggregated Ig was one of those factors that supported a monocytic lineage for HCs. Secondly, the non-specific binding of polyclonal Mabs, which caused diagnostic and experimental difficulties during the 1970s, is largely attributable to FCγRII activity.

HCs also express the principal 'lymphocyte homing receptors'. These molecules are less specific and are present on lymphocytes at a wide range of maturational stages. Lymphocyte selectin (L-selectin) is expressed by HCs as well as by a wide range of normal and malignant lymphocytes (A. Vincent, unpublished data). HCs also express the other major homing molecule, CD44 [214]. However, the function of non-integrin homing receptors has not specifically been studied in relation to HC biology.

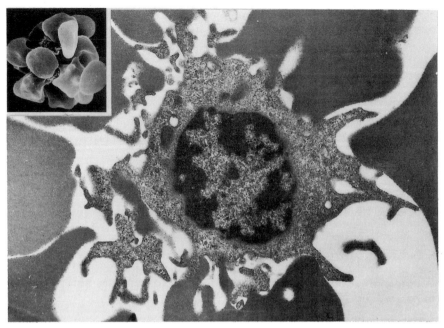

Fig. 7.11. γFc rosettes. Indicator erythrocytes make contact with the HCs over large areas and are markedly deformed by the process. (Inset) SEM of rosette.

7.8.2
Integrins

The integrin family of receptors has been a particular interest of the authors. The principal integrins expressed by HCs, together with their potential cellular functions, are given in Table 7.5 (reviewed in [50, 52]).

7.8.3
Adhesion molecules and HC behaviour

The resistance of HCs to cell killing by NK or LAK cells in *in vitro* assays has been implicated as an element in the survival of the malignant clone *in vivo*.The Ig superfamily adhesion molecule ICAM-1 and the leukocyte integrin LFA-1 (αLβ2) are important in immune recognition. Both molecules are present in limited amounts or are not expressed by HCs [193]. It has been suggested that the low level of expression of these two important adhesion molecules may be a significant factor in the lack of immune cell recognition of HCs and their consequent resistance to NK/LAK killing [193].

In terms of the tissue distribution of the malignant cells, integrins almost certainly play a major role. α4β1 is the dominant endothelial/cell binding integrin on HCs. The ligand of α4β1 is VCAM. Under normal conditions VCAM-1 is expressed only at limited sites, principally bone marrow stroma and splenic and hepatic sinusoids [322, 343]. These sites are the major areas of HC infiltration *in vivo*. Moreover, HCs are known to secrete TNFα. Since the cytokine strongly induces VCAM expression

Table 7.5 The principal integrin receptors expressed by hairy cells

Integrin	Principal ligand(s)	Amount	Comment
(i) Cell-binding integrins			
β2 integrins			
LFA-1 (αLβ2)	ICAM family	+/−	
MAC-1 (αMβ2)	ICAM-1, iC3b	+	Pattern of expression is an inversion of the usual pattern in B cells, where p150,95 is usually absent and LFA-1 predominates
p150,95 (αXβ2)	iC3b	+++	
α4 and β7 integrins			
VLA-4 (α4β1)	VCAM-1, (FN)	++	
α4β7	VCAM-1, (FN), MADCAM	0	Expression of α4β1 without α4β7 is unusual, and has been reported only on HCs and plasma cells. Expression of HML-1 is almost unique to HCs among B cells, although it is expressed on gut-associated T cells
HML-1 (αHβ7)	E-cadherin	++	
(ii) Adhesive protein-binding integrins			
β1 integrins			
VLA-4 (α4β1)	FN, (VCAM)	++	
VLA-5 (α5β1)	FN	+++	VLA-4 is widely expressed on B cells. However, VLA-5 is acquired by B cells only after activation *in vitro* or *in vivo*
αv integrins			
VNR (αvβ3)	VN (FN, Fb, TSP)	+	
αvβ1	FN	+	αv integrins are not normally expressed on B cells. On T cells they are acquired following activation

by endothelia [58], TNF-induced VCAM expression in HC-rich areas may serve to encourage further ingress of malignant cells.

The role of the other cell-binding integrins expressed by HCs is less clear. Both αMβ2 and αXβ2 recognise endothelial ligands [59], but are also important complement receptors (CR3 and CR4, respectively). The expression and activity of these complement-binding integrins may therefore play a role in the long-recognised 'monocytic' feature of HCs – the ability to phagocytose [136]. Similarly, although αHβ7 integrin is perhaps the most unique marker of HCs, its function on the malignant cell is unexplained. A ligand for αHβ7 (E-cadherin) has been described on epithelial cells [76]. However, present knowledge of the tissue distribution of E-cadherin does not identify a role for this molecule in the behaviour of HCs.

The adhesive-protein interactions mediated by integrins may also be very

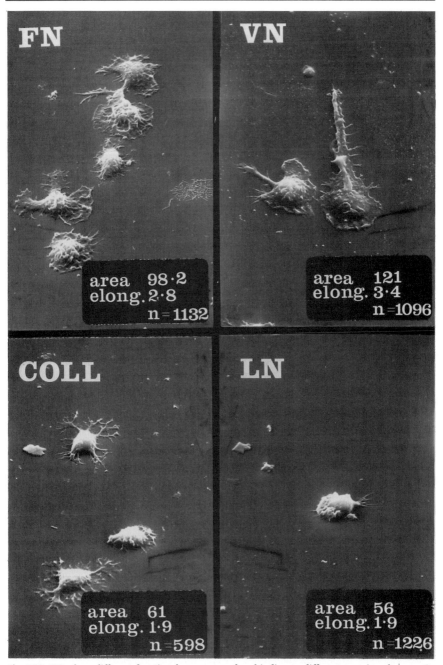

Fig. 7.12. HCs show different functional responses when binding to different protein substrata. On fibronectin (FN) HCs spread in a non-polar fashion, indicating strong adherence. On vitronectin (VN) spreading is polarised, which indicates cell motility. On collagen (COLL) and laminin (LN) HCs show a minimal, non-spreading (sessile) adhesion. The inset panels indicate the average spreading (area) and polarisation (elong, cell elongation) for the cell population (n).

important in HC biology (Fig. 7.12). In particular, the αvβ3 integrin appears to mediate HC motility. αvβ3 is increasingly recognised to have an important role in cell migration in general; for example, the acquisition of this integrin is an important feature determining the migratory (invasive) phenotype in malignant melanoma [314]. The principal ligand for αvβ3 is vitronectin (VN), a widely distributed adhesive protein that is particularly rich within splenic red pulp stroma [330]. In concert with the VCAM-rich splenic endothelium, VN may therefore function to promote the further ingress of circulating HCs into the splenic red pulp. A second adhesion receptor, that for hyaluronic acid, has also been reported to mediate HC motility [289]; how this receptor contributes to HC behaviour is still unclear.

Finally, we have suggested an important role for the α5β1 integrin [51]. HCs, like fibroblastic cells, are able to synthesise fibronectin (FN) and, through the action of α5β1 and a less well-defined 'matrix assembly site', are able to form a polymeric matrix of FN *in vitro*. We have suggested that this ability may partly underlie the bone marrow fibrosis characteristic of the disorder (Section 3.1).

7.9
Cell survival and cell death

The HC is not a rapidly proliferative cell (Fig. 7.13). The disease shows relatively slow clinical progress, and proliferating cells are rarely identified on *ex vivo* sections or

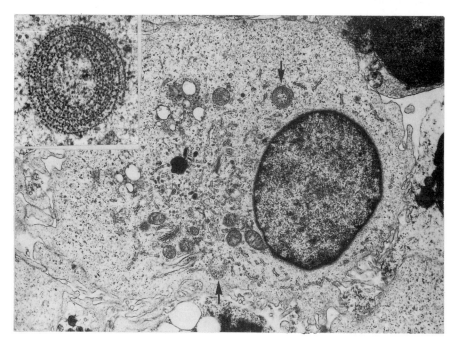

Fig. 7.13. A PHA-transformed HC blast. The cell contains two ribosome–lamellar complexes (arrows) and is presumably therefore derived from a hairy cell. The inset shows the typical features of the R–L complex. Such cells form only a minority of blast cells in stimulated HC preparations, the majority being derived from T cells.

blood/marrow smears. Similarly, spontaneous metaphases are very rare *in vitro*, and agents such as TNFα or BCGF that induce HC proliferation generally induce only low levels, detected not by an increase in the number of malignant cells but by radio-nucleotide incorporation or by the appearance of nuclear proliferation antigens [83, 113, 149]. Thus, although some *in vitro* proliferation systems can effectively induce metaphases and division of HCs [198, 212], it seems likely that abnormal cell survival rather than rapid proliferation underlies the abnormal accumulation of cells in HCL.

The mechanism of cell survival in HCL has received relatively little attention to date; however, some aspects have been addressed. HCs express bcl-2 protein and also express fas: both of these molecules have a role in apoptosis but the significance of their expression by HCs is unclear. It is, however, clear that HCs cultured *in vitro* die over a period of 3–10 days through spontaneous apoptosis. The cells show typical changes of apoptosis, namely, nuclear fragmentation, surface blebbing and loss of volume, together with characteristic DNA laddering on gel analysis. This cell survival is sensitive to a number of environmental factors, and is rapidly induced by addition of purine analogue drugs [61].

Appendix A: Tartrate-resistant acid phosphatase (TRAP)

Consistent cytochemical demonstration of TRAP in HCs requires attention to several technical factors, which have been carefully reviewed by Janckila *et al.* [183].

The method recommended by these authors for smears of blood and marrow is given below. The sensitivity of the reaction is determined by the coupler used: fast garnet GBC produces maximum sensitivity and is recommended for the demonstration of TRAP in peripheral blood HCs. Hexasotised pararosaniline as coupler is less sensitive and is therefore not optimal for peripheral blood smears. However, the specific fine reaction produced by pararosaniline makes it suitable for histological sections and dab preparations, where fast garnet GBC frequently gives non-specific precipitates.

Reagents

1. *Fixative (buffered methanol–acetone)* Add 10 ml methanol and 60 ml acetone to 30 ml aqueous solution containing 0.63 g citric acid (final citrate concentration, 0.03 M). Mix well. Adjust the pH of this mixture to 5.4 with concentrated NaOH solution. Store at 4–10 °C. Shake before use. This fixative is stable for at least a month.
2. *Stock substrate solution:* Dissolve 100 mg naphthol ASBI phosphoric acid in 10 ml N-N dimethylformamide. Store at 4–10 °C in a glass-capped bottle in the dark. This solution is stable for two to three months, or until it turns pink.
3. *Acetate buffer (0.1 N, pH 5.2):* Dissolve 13.6 g sodium acetate trihydrate in distilled water to make 1 litre (Solution A). Dilute 6.0 ml glacial acetic acid to 1 litre with distilled water (Solution B). Titrate Solution A to pH 5.2 with Solution B. Store at 4–10 °C to retard fungal growth. This solution is stable for at least three months.
4. *Acetate–tartrate buffer (0.05 M tartrate in 0.1 N acetate buffer, final pH 5.2):* Dissolve 3.75 g pf L(+) tartaric acid in 490 ml of 0.1 N acetate buffer. Adjust pH to 5.2 with concentrated NaOH solution. Bring volume to 500 ml with distilled water. Store at 4–10 °C. The solution is stable for at least three months.
5. *Mayer's haematoxylin:* Self-prepared or purchased from commercial source.
6. *Glycerine jelly:* Self-prepared or purchased from commercial source.
7. *Fast garnet GBC*

Staining procedure

1. Fix smears with cold, buffered methanol–acetone fixative for 30 seconds. Wash 5–6 times with distilled water. Air dry.

2. Incubate smears at 37 °C in the following medium for 45-60 minutes:
   Acetate-tartrate buffer: 50 ml
   Stock substrate solution:1 ml
   Fast garnet GBC salt: 25 mg
   Filter the incubating solution before use.
1. Wash smears with water. Counterstain with Mayer's haematoxylin for 1-5 minutes.
2. Wash in running tap water for 5-10 minutes.
3. Dry thoroughly and mount in glycerine jelly.

Interpretation

Strong TRAP positivity must be present in the abnormal mononuclear cells to support the diagnosis of HCL; the neutrophils in the same preparation must lack enzyme activity. Weak staining may occur in other lymphoproliferative disorders and is therefore not diagnostic (Section 7.2.1). When the above method is used, TRAP is demonstrable in virtually all cases. Genuinely negative cases of true HCL are exceptionally rare but probably do occur.

Notes

Controls If the putative HCs possess strong TRAP while adjacent neutrophils are negative, then further controls barely matter. If, however, the abnormal mononuclear cells are negative, then a positive control smear of HCL is required. A negative control is not really necessary providing the neutrophils in the preparation are clearly negative. Similarly, although often recommended, a control omitting tartrate serves little purpose. A reasonable routine, therefore, is simply to include a known HCL smear as a positive control for the full TRAP stain.

Storage of control material Positive control slides should be fixed and then stored in metal foil in a refrigerator; material prepared in this way retains enzyme activity for a prolonged period (years). Unfixed slides stored at room temperature retain activity for at least 4 weeks.

Appendix B: CD-antigen expression by HCs

Antigen	Exp	Name/function
CD1A	+	Restricted presentation to T cells
CD1B	0	Restricted presentation to T cells
CD1C	0	Restricted presentation to T cells
CD2	0	CD58 ligand (immune-cell adhesion)
CD3	0	Associated with T-cell receptor complex
CD4	0	Accessory molecule in MHC recognition
CD5	±	CD72 ligand (?), TCR accessory molecule, activation or lineage-specific marker on B cells
CD6		?Signalling in T (and B) cells
CD7		Early T-cell marker, ? signals
CD8	0	Accessory molecule in MHC recognition
CD9	+	Induces Fc-receptor-dependent activation in various cell types
CD10	±	Neutral endopeptidase
CD11a (int)	±	Integrin: LFA1
CD11b (int)	+	Integrin: Mac 1
CD11c (int)	+++	Integrin: p150,95
CD12	0	?
CD13	0	Aminopeptidase
CD14	0	LPS receptor
CD15	0	Sialylated Lewis X, CD62 ligand
CD16	0	FcγRIII (low affinity Ig receptor)
CD17	0	Lactosylceramide
CD18 (int)	+++	Integrin: β2 family subunit
CD19	++	Part of B-cell signalling complex
CD20	+++	Calcium channel in B-cell activation
CD21	0	Part of B-cell signalling complex
CD22	+++	Adhesion molecule involved in B-cell activation
		CD23+Regulation of IgE response
CD24	+	?
CD25	++	IL2-receptor α-subunit
CD26	+	Serine exopeptidase
CD27 (TNF)		?Signalling (CD70 ligand)
CD28		B-cell activation, ? signalling
CD29 (int)	+++	Integrin: β1 family subunit
CD30 (TNF)	0	Receptor for unknown cytokine on B and T cells
CD31	++	PECAM, involved in transmigration

Antigen	Exp	Name/function
CD32	++	FcγRII receptor
CD33	0	?(Myeloid precursor marker)
CD34	0	? (Immature haemopoietic precursors and endothelial cells)
CD35	0	Complement receptor 1
CD36	+	Thrombospondin receptor (and other functions)
CD37	+++	?Function (B-cell marker)
CD38	+	?(Present on activated B and T cells)
CD39	++	?
CD40 (TNF)	+++	? Involved in selection process in B-cell germinal centres.
CD41 (int)	0	Integrin: αIIb
CD42a,b,c,d	0	VWF receptor complex
CD43	+	Involved in adhesion
CD44	++	Matrix binding and homing molecule
CD45	+++	Leukocyte common antigen (phosphotyrosine phosphatase)
CD46		Complement binding protein
CD47	++	Widespread distribution, ? involved in cation flux
CD48		Counter receptor for CD2 in mouse
CD49a (int)	±	Integrin: α1
CD49b (int)	0	Integrin: α2
CD49c (int)	±	Integrin: α3
CD49d (int)	++	Integrin: α4
CD49e (int)	+++	Integrin: α5
CD49f (int)	0	Integrin: α6
CD50		ICAM-3 (LFA-1 receptor)
CD51 (int)	+	Integrin: αv
CD52		Campath-1
CD53		Tetraspan family ? function
CD54	±	ICAM-1 (LFA-1 receptor)
CD55		Limits complement activation
CD56		N-CAM (homotypic adhesion)
CD57		?Function (NK- and T-cell marker)
CD58		Counter receptor for CD2
CD59		Counter receptor for CD2
CD60		Augments CD3 signal
CD61	+	Integrin: β3 chain
CD62E	0	E-selectin
CD62L	++	L-selectin
CD62P	0	P-selectin
CD63		?(Activated platelet marker)
CD64	0	FcγR1 (monomeric Ig receptor)
CD65	0	Ceramide dodecasaccharide 4c
CD66a,b,c	0	?(BGP, p100, CEA)
CD68	+	?(Lysosomal membrane components)

Antigen	Exp	Name/function
CD69	0	Early lymphocyte activation
CD70		CD27 ligand
CD71	++	Transferrin receptor
CD72	++	?CD5 ligand
CD73	0	Catalyses dephosphorylation of ribonucleotides
CD74	+++	Associates with and transports class II molecules
CDw75	+++	?
CDw76	+++	?
CD77	0	Possible role in apoptosis
CD78	+	Role in IgM-induced B-cell proliferation
CD79a,b		B-cell receptor components
CD80		B7/BB1 CD28 ligand, involved in T-cell activation
CD81		TAPA1, B-cell-signalling with CD19 and CD21
CD82		?Signal transduction
CD83		On DRCs and activated lymphocytes (? antigen presentation)
CDw84		?
CD85	+++	? Function (widespread reactivity on B cells and plasma cells)
CD86		Activation antigen on B cells
CD87		UPA-R
CD88		C5aR
CD89		FCαR
CDw90		?(Expressed principally on immature haemopoietic cells)
CD91		α2-macroglobulin receptor
CDw92		Granulo-monocytic antigen and on PBLs, ? function
CD93		Granulo-monocytic antigen, ? function
CD94		Acts in integrin-mediated adhesion of NK cells
CD95	++	FAS antigen, APO-1, mediates apoptosis
CD96		Tactile (T-cell activation, increased late expression)
CD97		Activation antigen on B and T cells, ? function
CD98		Associates with CD45, ? function
CD99/CD99R		Adhesion, particularly T and NK cells
CD100		B-cell activation antigen
CDw101		?Related to CD28 function in T cells
CD102		ICAM-2 (ligand for LFA-1)
CD103 (int)	++	αH integrin chain
CD104 (int)	0	β4 integrin chain
CD105		Endoglin, ? function
CD106	+	VCAM (VLA-4 integrin ligand)
CD107a,b		LAMP1 and 2 (lysosome-associated membrane proteins)

Antigen	Exp	Name/function
CDw108	++	?Developmentally regulated expression on B cells
CDw109		?Accessory molecule in lymphocyte activation
CD115	++	M-CSFR (CSF-1R)
CDw116	++	GM-CSFR
CD117		Stem cell factor receptor (c-kit)
CDw119	++	IFNγR
CD120a,b	++	TNFR (p55 and p75)
CDw121a,b		IL-1R (types 1 and 2)
CD122	+	IL-2R β chain
CDw124		IL-4R
CD126	+	IL-6R
CDw127		IL-7R
CDw128		IL-8R
CDw130	+	IL-GR

Sources: [214, 320]; other references as in Chapters 4 and 7.

(TNF), TNF receptor family; (int), integrin family.

No symbol, not determined; 0, not expressed; $\pm$, very low level expression or expressed on few cases only; +, low level or variable low-moderate expression; ++, consistent moderate expression; +++, strong expression.

References

1. Abbondanzo SL, Sulak LE: Ki-1-positive lymphoma developing 10 years after the diagnosis of hairy cell leukemia. Cancer 67(12):3117, 1991
2. Adami F, Chilosi M, Lestani M, Scarpa A, Zambello R, Pomponi F, Semenzato G, Menestrina F: A CD5+ leukemic lymphoma with monocytoid features: an unusual B-cell lymphoma mimicking hairy-cell leukemia. Acta Haematol 89(2):94, 1993
3. Aderem A: Signal transduction and the actin cytoskeleton: the roles of MARKS and profilin. TIBS 17:438, 1992
4. Aderka D, Michalevicz R, Daniel Y, Levo Y, Douer D, Ben-Bassat I, Ramot B, Shaklai M, Prokocimer M, Berrebi A, et al.: Recombinant interferon alpha-C for advanced hairy cell leukemia. An Israeli multicenter study. Cancer 61(11):2207, 1988
5. Aksoy M: Chronic lymphoid leukemia and hairy-cell leukemia due to chronic exposure to benzene – report of 3 cases. Brit J Haematol 66(2):209, 1987
6. Aljurf M, Cornbleet PJ, Michel F: CD5+ chronic B-cell leukemia with features intermediate to chronic lymphocytic leukemia and hairy cell leukemia. Hematol Pathol 8(3):99, 1994
7. Al-Katib A, Wang CY, McKenzie S, Clarkson BD, Koziner B: Phorbol ester-induced hairy cell features on chronic lymphocytic leukemia cells in vitro. Am J Hematol 40(4):264, 1992
8. Al-Katib A, Mohammad RM, Dan M, Hussein ME, Akhtar A, Pettit GR, Sensenbrenner LL: Bryostatin 1-induced hairy cell features on chronic lymphocytic leukemia cells in vitro. Exp Hematol 21(1):61, 1993
9. Ambrus JL Jr, Chesky L, McFarland P, Young KR Jr, Mostowski H, August A, Chused TM: Induction of proliferation by high molecular weight B cell growth factor or low molecular weight B cell growth factor is associated with increases in intracellular calcium in different subpopulations of human B lymphocytes. Cell Immunol 134(2):314, 1991
10. Anday G, Goodman JR, Tishkoff GH: An unusual cytoplasmic ribososmal structure in pathological lymphocytes. Blood 41:439, 1973
11. Anderson KC, Boyd AW, Fisher DC, Leslie D, Schlossman SF, Nadler LM: Hairy-cell leukemia – a tumor of pre-plasma cells. Blood 65(3):620, 1985
12. Annino L, Ferrari A, Giona F, Cimino G, Crescenzi S, Cava MC, Pacchiarotti A, Mandelli F: Deoxycoformycin induces long-lasting remissions in hairy cell leukemia: clinical and biological results of two different regimens. Leuk Lymphoma 14 (suppl 1):115, 1994
13. Antonelli G, Dianzani F: Antibodies to interferon in patients. Arch Virol 8 (suppl):271, 1993
14. Arai E, Ikeda S, Itoh S, Katayama I: Specific skin lesions as the presenting symptom of hairy cell leukemia. Am J Clin Pathol 90(4):459, 1988
15. Arena FP: Treatment of hairy cell leukemia in a decade of change. Appraisal of community based oncologists' opinions. Leuk Lymphoma 14 (suppl 1):85, 1994
16. Armitage RJ, Worman CP, Galvin MC, Cawley JC: Hairy-cell leukemia with hybrid B-T features – a study with a panel of monoclonal antibodies. Am J Hematol 18(4):335, 1985
17. Armitage RJ, Macduff BM, Eisenman J, Paxton R, Grabstein KH: Interleukin 15 has stimulatory activity for the induction of B cell proliferation and differentiation. J Immunol 154:483, 1995
18. Barak V, Nisman B, Dann EJ, Kalickman I, Ruchlemer R, Bennett MA, Polliack A: Serum interleukin 1 beta levels as a marker in hairy cell leukemia: correlation with disease status and sIL-2R levels. Leuk Lymphoma 14 (suppl 1):33, 1994
19. Barbara JA, Smith WB, GambleJR, Van Ostacle X, Tavernier J, Fiers W, Vadas MA, Lopez AF: Dissociation of TNF alpha cytotoxic and proinflammatory activities by p55 receptor- and p75 receptor-selective TNF alpha mutants. Embo J 843, 1994
20. Barut BA, Cochran MK, O'Hara C, Anderson KC: Response patterns of hairy cell leukemia to B-cell mitogens and growth factors. Blood 76(10):2091, 1990

21. Barut B, Chauhan D, Uchiyama H, Anderson KC: Interleukin-6 functions as an intracellular growth factor in hairy cell leukemia *in vitro*. J Clin Invest 92(5):2346, 1993
22. Begley CG, Burton JD, Tsudo M, Brownstein BH, Ambrus JL, Walman TA: Human B lymphocytes express the p75 component of the human IL-2 receptor. Leuk Res 14:263, 1990
23. Bentz M, Dohner H, Guckel F, Semmler W, Kauczor HU, van-Kaick G, Ho AD, Hunstein W: Assessment of bone marrow infiltration by magnetic resonance imaging in patients with hairy cell leukemia treated with pentostatin or alpha-interferon. Leukemia 5(10):905, 1991
24. Berman E, Heller G, Kempin S, Gee T, Tran LL, Clarkson B: Incidence of response and long-term follow-up in patients with hairy cell leukemia treated with recombinant interferon alfa-2a [see comments]. Blood 75(4):839, 1990
25. Bernstein L, Newton P, Ross RK: Epidemiology of hairy cell leukemia in Los Angeles County. Cancer Res 50(12):3605, 1990
26. Berrebi A, Bassous-Guedj L, Vorst E, Dagan S, Shtalrid M, Freedman A: Further characterization of prolymphocytic leukemia cells as a tumor of activated B cells [see comments]. Am J Hematol 34(3):181, 1990
27. Betticher DC, Fey MF, von-Rohr A, Tobler A, Jenzer H, Gratwohl A, Lohri A, Pugin P, Hess U, Pagani O, *et al.*: High incidence of infections after 2-chlorodeoxyadenosine (2-CDA) therapy in patients with malignant lymphomas and chronic and acute leukaemias. Ann Oncol 5(1):57, 1994
28. Bianchi AC, Heslop HE, Drexler HG, Cordingley FT, Turner M, De-Mel WC, Hoffbrand AV, Brenner MK: Effects of tumour necrosis factor and alpha interferon on chronic B cell malignancies. Nouv Rev Fr Hematol 30(5/6):317, 1988
29. Billard C, Ferbus D, Sigaux F, Castaigne S, Degos L, Flandrin G, Falcoff E: Action of interferon-alpha on hairy cell leukemia: expression of specific receptors and (2'-5')oligo (A) synthetase in tumor cells from sensitive and resistant patients. Leuk Res 12(1):11, 1988
30. Billard C, Sigaux F, Wietzerbin J: IFN-alpha *in vivo* enhances tumor necrosis factor receptor levels on hairy cells. J Immunol 145(6):1713, 1990
31. Billard C, Lasfar A: Production of tumor necrosis factor in response to interferon-alpha in hairy cell leukemia [letter; comment]. Leukemia 7(2):331, 1993
32. Blum SF: Lithium in hairy cell leukemia. N Engl J Med 303:464, 1980
33. Bouroncle BA, Wiseman BK, Doan CA: Leukemic reticuloendotheliosis. Blood 13:609, 1958
34. Bouroncle BA: Unusual presentations and complications of hairy cell leukemia. Leukemia 1:288, 1987
35. Bouroncle BA: Thirty-five years in the progress of hairy cell leukemia. Leuk Lymphoma 14 (suppl 1):1, 1994
36. Bouza E, Burgaleta C, Golde DW: Infections in hairy cell leukemia. Blood 51:851, 1978
37. Branda RF: Leukemic reticuloendotheliosis and 'hairy cells'. N Engl J Med 295:1015, 1976
38. Bray D, White JG: Cortical flow in animal cells. Science 239:883, 1988
39. Braylan RC, Jaffe ES, Triche TJ, Namba K, Fowlkes BJ, Metzger H, Frank MM, Dolan MS, Yee CL, Green I, Berard CW: Structural and functional properties of the 'hairy cells' of leukemic reticuloendotheliosis. Cancer 41:210, 1978
40. Brito-Babapulle V, Ellis J, Matutes E, Oscier D, Khokhar T, MacLennan K, Catovsky D: Translocation t(11;14)(q13;q32) in chronic lymphoid disorders. Genes Chromosom Cancer 5(2):158, 1992
41. Brogden RN, Sorkin EM: Pentostatin. A review of its pharmacodynamic and pharmacokinetic properties, and therapeutic potential in lymphoproliferative disorders. Drugs 46(4):652, 1993
42. Bryson HM, Sorkin EM: Cladribine. A review of its pharmacodynamic and pharmacokinetic properties and therapeutic potential in haematological malignancies. Drugs 46(5):872, 1993
43. Buck C, Digel W, Schoniger W, Stefanic M, Ragnavachar A, Heimpel H, Porzsolt F: Tumor necrosis factor-alpha, but not lymphotoxin, stimulates growth of tumor cells in hairy cell leukemia. Leukemia 4(6):431, 1990
44. Burke JS, Byrne GE, Rappaport H: Hairy cell leukemia (leukemic reticulondotheliosis). A clinical pathologic study of 21 patients. Cancer 33:2267, 1974
45. Burke JS: The value of the bone-marrow in the diagnosis of hairy cell leukemia. Am J Clin Pathol 70:876, 1978
46. Burns GF, Flemens RJ, Barker CR, Cawley JC, Worman CP, Hayhoe FGJ: Leukemic reticuloendotheliosis and 'hairy cells'. N Engl J Med 295:1015, 1976
47. Burns GF, Cawley JC, Higgy KE, Barker CR, Edwards M, Rees JKH, Hayhoe FJG: Hairy cell leukaemia: a B cell neoplasm with a severe deficency of circulating normal B lymphocytes. Leuk Res 2:33, 1978

48. Burns GF, Cawley JC, Worman CP, Karpas A, Barker CR, Goldstone AH, Hayhoe FGJ: Multiple heavy chain isotypes on the surface of the cells of hairy-cell leukaemia. Blood 52:1132, 1978
49. Burthem J, Baker PK, Hunt JA, Cawley JC: The function of c-fms in hairy-cell leukemia: macrophage colony-stimulating factor stimulates hairy-cell movement. Blood 83(5):1381, 1994
50. Burthem J, Baker PK, Hunt JA, Cawley JC: Hairy cell interactions with extracellular matrix: expression of specific integrin receptors and their role in the cell's response to specific adhesive proteins. Blood 84(3):873, 1994
51. Burthem J, Cawley JC: The bone marrow fibrosis of hairy-cell leukemia is caused by the synthesis and assembly of a fibronectin matrix by the hairy cells. Blood 83(2):497, 1994
52. Burthem J, Cawley JC: Specific tissue invasion, localisation and matrix modification in hairy-cell leukemia. Leuk Lymphoma 14 (suppl 1):19, 1994
53. Burton J, Kay NE: Does IL-2 receptor expression and secretion in chronic B-cell leukemia have a role in down-regulation of the immune system? Leukemia 8(1):92, 1994
54. Caldwell CW, Patterson WP: Relationship between CD45 antigen expression and putative stages of differentiation in B-cell malignancies. Am J Hematol 36(2):111, 1991
55. Caligaris-Cappio FG, Bergui L, Corbascio G, Tousco F, Marchisio PC: Cytoskeletal organisation is aberrantly rearranged in the cells of B chronic lymphocytic leukemia. Blood 67:233, 1986
56. Capnist G, Federico M, Chisesi T, Resegotti L, Pagnucco G, Castoldi GL, Lamparelli T, Frassoldati A, Guarnaccia C, Leoni P, et al.: Should alpha interferon be used as primary treatment for hairy cell leukemia? Italian Cooperative Group for Hairy Cell Leukemia. Leuk Res 15(6):419, 1991
57. Capnist G, Federico M, Chisesi T, Resegotti L, Lamparelli T, Fabris P, Rossi G, Invernizzi R, Guarnaccia C, Leoni P, et al.: Long term results of interferon treatment in hairy cell leukemia. Italian Cooperative Group for Hairy Cell Leukemia (ICGHCL). Leuk Lymphoma 14(5/6):457, 1994
58. Carlos TM, Schwartz BR, Kovach NL, Yee E, Rosso M, Osborn L, Chi-Rosso G, Newman B, Lobb R, Harlan JM: Vascular cell adhesion molecule-1 mediates lymphocyte adherence to cytokine-activated cultured human endothelial cells. Blood 76:965, 1990
59. Carlos TM, Harlan JM: Leukocyte–endothelial adhesion molecules. Blood 84:2068, 1994
60. Carrera MD, Saven A, Piro LD: Purine metabolism of lymphocytes. Targets for chemotherapy drug development. New Drug Therapy 8:357, 1994
61. Carson DA, Carrera CJ, Wasson DB, Yamanaka H: Programmed cell death and adenine deoxynucleotide metabolism in human lymphocytes. Adv Enzyme Regul 27:395, 1988
62. Carson DA, Wasson DB, Esparza LM, Carrera CJ, Kipps TJ, Cottam HB: Oral antilymphocyte activity and induction of apoptosis by 2-chloro-2'-arabino-fluoro-2'-deoxyadenosine. Proc Natl Acad Sci USA 89(7):2970, 1992
63. Castaigne S, Sigaux F, Degos L, Flandrin G: Hairy cell leukemia: follow-up after completion of alpha interferon treatment. Nouv Rev Fr Hematol 31(5):321, 1989
64. Castro-Malaspina H, Najean Y, Flandrin G: Erythrokinetic studies in hairy cell leukaemia. Brit J Haematol 42:189, 1979
65. Catovsky D, Pettit JE, Galton DAG, Spiers ASD, Harrison CV: Leukaemic reticuloendotheliosis ('hairy cell leukaemia'): a distinct clinico-pathological entity. Brit J Haematol 26:9, 1974
66. Catovsky D: Hairy cell leukaemia and prolymphocytic leukaemia. Clin Haematol 6:245, 1977
67. Catovsky D: Prolymphocytic and hairy cell leukaemias, in Gunz F, Henderson ES (eds): Leukemia (4th edn). New York, Grune and Stratton, 1982, p 759
68. Catovsky D, Costello C, Loukopoulus D: Hairy cell leukaemia and myelomatosis: Chance association or clinical manefestations of the same B-cell disease spectrum? Blood 57:758, 1981
69. Catovsky D, Obrien M, Melo JV, Wardle J, Brozovic M: Hairy-cell leukemia (hcl) variant – an intermediate disease between hcl and b prolymphocytic leukemia. Semin Oncol 11(4):362, 1984
70. Catovsky D, Golomb HM, Golde DW: General commentary on the Second International Workshop. Leukemia 1:407, 1987
71. Catovsky D, Foa R, eds: The Lymphoid Leukaemias: The Leukaemic Phase of Non-Hodgkins Lymphoma. London, Butterworths, 1990
72. Catovsky D, Matutes E, Talavera JG, O'Connor NT, Johnson SA, Emmett E, Corbett L, Swansbury J: Long term results with 2'-deoxycoformycin in hairy cell leukemia. Leuk Lymphoma 14 (suppl 1):109, 1994
73. Cawley JC, Burns GF, Hayhoe FGH, eds: Hairy-Cell Leukaemia. Heidleberg, Springer, 1980
74. Cawley JC, Burns GF, Hayhoe FGJ: A chronic lymphoproliferative disorder with distinctive features – a distinct variant of hairy-cell leukemia. Leuk Res 4(6):547, 1980

75. Cawley JC, Burns GF, Worman CP, Roberts BE, Hayhoe FGJ: Clinical and haematological fluctuations in hairy cell leukaemia: sequential surface-marker analysis. Blood 55:784, 1980
76. Cepek KL, Shaw SK, Parker CM, Russel GJ, Morrow JS, Rimm DL, Brenner MB: Adhesion between epithelial cells and T lymphocytes mediated by E-cadherin and the alpha E beta 7 integrin. Nature 372:190, 1994
77. Chang KL, Chen YY, Weiss LM: Lack of evidence of Epstein–Barr virus in hairy cell leukemia and monocytoid B-cell lymphoma. Hum Pathol 24(1):58, 1993
78. Cheever MA, Fefer A, Greenberg PD, Appelbaum F, Armitge JD, Buchner CD, Sale GE, Witherspoon RP, Thomas ED: Treatment of hairy cell leukemia with chemo-radio-therapy and identical twin bone marrow transplantation. N Engl J Med 307:479, 1992
79. Child JA, Cawley JC, Martin S, Ghoneim ATM: Microbicidal function of the neutrophils in hairy-cell leukaemia. Acta Haematol 62:191, 1978
80. Cimino G, Annino L, Giona F, Sgadari C, Di-Gregorio AO, Cava MC, Cimino G, Mandelli F: Serum interleukin-1 beta levels correlate with neoplastic bulk in hairy cell leukemia. Leukemia 5(7):602, 1991
81. Cogliatti SB, Lennert K, Hansmann ML, Zwingers TL: Monocytoid B cell lymphoma: clinical and prognostic features of 21 patients. J Clin Pathol 43:619, 1990
82. Cohen A, Thompson E: DNA repair in nondividing human lymphocytes: inhibition by deoxyadenosine. Cancer Res 46:1585, 1986
83. Cordingley FT, Bianchi A, Hoffbrand AV, Reittie JE, Heslop HE, Vyakarnam A, Turner M, Meager A, Brenner MK: Tumour necrosis factor as an autocrine tumour growth factor for chronic B-cell malignancies. Lancet 1(8592):969, 1988
84. Cordingley FT, Hoffbrand AV, Brenner MK: Cytokine-induced enhancement of the susceptibility of hairy cell leukaemia lymphocytes to natural killer cell lysis. Brit J Haematol 70(1):37, 1988
85. Cordonnier C, Farcet JP, Desforges L, Brunbuisson C, Vernant JP, Kuentz M, Dournon E: Legionnaires-disease and hairy-cell leukaemia – an unfortuitous association. Arch Intern Med 144(12):2373, 1984
86. Dalri P, Boi S, Cristofolini M, Piscioli F, Rubertelli M: Sweet syndrome – presenting symptom of hairy-cell leukaemia with fatal infection by pneumocy tis-carinii. Haematologica 67(5):765, 1982
87. Damasio EE, Frassoldati A: Splenectomy following complete response to alpha interferon (IFN) therapy in patients with hairy cell leukemia (HCL): results of the HCL88 protocol. Italian Cooperative Group for Hairy Cell Leukemia (ICGHCL). Leuk Lymphoma 14 (suppl 1):95, 1994
88. Daniel MT, Flandarin G: Fine structure of abnormal cells in hairy cell leukemia, with special reference to their *in vitro* phagocytic ability. Lab Invest 30:1, 1974
89. Davis TE, Waterbury L, Abelhoff M, Burke PJ: Leukemic reticuloendotheliosis. Report of a case with prolonged remission following intensive chemotherapy. Arch Intern Med 136:620, 1976
90. Delsol G, Pelligrin M, Corberand J, Guiu M, Pris J, Fabre J: Kupffer Cells and Other Liver Sinusoidal Cells. Amsterdam, Elsevier, 1977
91. Demeter J, Paloczi K, Foldi J, Hokland M, Hokland P, Benczur M, Lehoczky D: Immunological and molecular biological identification of a true case of T-hairy cell leukaemia. Eur J Haematol 43(4):339, 1989
92. Demeter J, Paloczi K, Lehoczky D, Benczur M: Hairy cell leukaemia: observations on natural killer activity in different clinical stages of the disease. Brit J Haematol 71(2):239, 1989
93. Demeter J, Grotes HJ, Horvath C, Gassel WD, Delling G, Friedrich JM, Porzsolt F: Bone densitometry and histomorphometry in patients with hairy cell leukemia. Leuk Lymphoma 14 (suppl 1):73, 1994
94. de-Totero D, Carbone A, Tazzari PL, Raspadori D, Ventura A, Reato G, Lauria F, Foa R: Expression of the IL2 receptor alpha, beta and gamma chains in hairy cell leukemia. Leuk Lymphoma 14 (suppl 1):27, 1994
95. di-Celle PF, Reato G, Raspadori D, Carbone A, Rondelli D, Lauria F, Foa R: Molecular evaluation of clonal remission in hairy cell leukemia patients treated with 2-chlorodeoxyadenosine. Leuk Lymphoma 14 (suppl 1):139, 1994
96. Digel W, Porzsolt F, Schmid M, Herrmann F, Lesslauer W, Brockhaus M: High levels of circulating soluble receptors for tumor necrosis factor in hairy cell leukemia and type B chronic lymphocytic leukemia. J Clin Invest 89(5):1690, 1992
97. Domingo A, Crespo N, Fernandez-de-Sevilla A, Domenech P, Jordan C, Callis M: Hairy cell leukemia and autoimmune hemolytic anemia. Leukemia 6(6):606, 1992
98. Drexler HG, Brenner MK, Gignac SM, Hoffbrand AV: Expression of tartrate-resistant acid

phosphatase in B-CLL treated with phorbol ester or phorbol ester plus calcium ionophore. Eur J Haematol 41(3):250, 1988

99. Drexler HG, Gignac SM: Characterization and expression of tartrate-resistant acid phosphatase (TRAP) in hematopoietic cells. Leukemia 8(3):359, 1994

100. Ellison DJ, Sharpe RW, Robbins BA, Spinosa JC, Leopard JD, Saven A, Piro LD: Immunomorphologic analysis of bone marrow biopsies after treatment with 2-chlorodeoxyadenosine for hairy cell leukemia. Blood 84(12):4310, 1994

101. Emberger JM, Navarro M, Rizkilla N, Izarn P: Splenic pseudosinuses, hepatic angiomatous lesions and hairy-cell leukemia. Am J Clin Pathol 69:194, 1973

102. Estey EH, Kurzrock R, Kantarjian HM, O'Brien SM, McCredie KB, Beran M, Koller C, Keating MJ, Hirsch-Ginsberg C, Huh YO, et al.: Treatment of hairy cell leukemia with 2-chlorodeoxyadenosine (2-CdA). Blood 79(4):882, 1992

103. Evans SS, Wang WC, Gregorio CC, Han T, Repasky EA: Interferon-alpha alters spectrin organization in normal and leukemic human B lymphocytes. Blood 81(3):759, 1993

104. Falini B, Pileri SA, Flenghi L, Liberati M, Stein H, Gerli R, Minelli O, Martelli MF, Lauria F, Poggi S: Selection of a panel of monoclonal antibodies for monitoring residual disease in peripheral blood and bone marrow of interferon-treated hairy cell leukaemia patients. Brit J Haematol 76(4):460, 1990

105. Farcet JP, Weschler J, Wirquin V, Divine M, Reyes F: Vasculitis in hairy-cell leukemia. Arch Intern Med 147(4):660, 1987

106. Fay JW, Moore JO, Logue JL, Huang AT: Lekopheresis therapy of leukemic reticuloendotheliosis. Blood 57:747, 1979

107. Federico M, Frassoldati A, Lamparelli T, Foa R, Brugiatelli M, Annino L, Baldini L, Capnist G, Chisesi T, di-Celle PF, et al.: Long-term results of alpha interferon as initial therapy and splenectomy as consolidation therapy in patients with hairy cell leukemia. Final report from the Italian Cooperative Group for HCL. Ann Oncol 5(8):725, 1994

108. Ferro LM, Zola H: Modulation of expression of the antigen identified by FMC7 upon human B-lymphocyte activation: evidence for differences between activation in vivo and in vitro. Immunology 69(3):373, 1990

109. Filleul B, Delannoy A, Ferrant A, Zenebergh A, Van-Daele S, Bosly A, Doyen C, Mineur P, Glorieux P, Driesschaert P, et al.: A single course of 2-chloro-deoxyadenosine does not eradicate leukemic cells in hairy cell leukemia patients in complete remission. Leukemia 8(7):1153, 1994

110. Flandrin G, Collado S: Is male predominance (4/1) in hairy-cell leukemia related to occupational exposure to ionizing-radiation, benzene and other solvents. Brit J Haematol 67(1):119, 1987

111. Foa R, Massaia M, Cardona S, Tos AG, Bianchi A, Attisano C, Guarini A, di-Celle PF, Fierro MT: Production of tumor necrosis factor-alpha by B-cell chronic lymphocytic leukemia cells: a possible regulatory role of TNF in the progression of the disease. Blood 76(2):393, 1990

112. Foa R, Guarini A, di-Celle PF, Trentin L, Gillio-Tos A, Bellone G, Carbone A, Attisano C, Massaia M, Raspadori D, et al.: Constitutive production of tumor necrosis factor-alpha in hairy cell leukemia: possible role in the pathogenesis of the cytopenia(s) and effect of treatment with interferon-alpha. J Clin Oncol 10(6):954, 1992

113. Ford RJ, Yoshimura L, Morgan J, Quesada J, Montagna R, Maizel A: Growth factor-mediated tumour cell proliferation in hairy-cell leukemia. J Exp Med 162:1093, 1985

114. Ford RJ, Kwok D, Quesada J, Sahasrabuddhe CG: Producion of B cell growth factor(s) by neoplastic hairy-cell leukemia patients. Blood 67:573, 1986

115. Frassoldati A, Lamparelli T, Federico M, Annino L, Capnist G, Pagnucco G, Dini E, Resegotti L, Damasio EE, Silingardi V: Hairy cell leukemia: a clinical review based on 725 cases of the Italian Cooperative Group (ICGHCL). Italian Cooperative Group for Hairy Cell Leukemia. Leuk Lymphoma 13(3/4):307, 1994

116. Galton JE, Bedford P, Scott JE, Brand CM, Nethersell AB: Antibodies to lymphoblastoid interferon [letter]. Lancet 2(8662):572, 1989

117. Galvani DW, Cawley JC: The current status of interferon alpha in haemic malignancy. Blood Rev 4:175, 1990

118. Gamliel H, Gurfel D, Wu SH, Golomb HM: Interferon-induced surface alterations in hairy cells. A review. Scanning Microsc 2(1):485, 1988

119. Gamliel H, Brownstein BH, Gurfel D, Wu SH, Rosner MC, Golomb HM: B-cell growth factor-induced and alpha-interferon-inhibited proliferation of hairy cells coincides with modulation of cell surface antigens. Cancer Res 50(13):4111, 1990

120. Ganeshaguru K, de-Mel WC, Sissolak G, Catovsky D, Dearden CE, Mehta AB, Hoffbrand AV: Increase in 2',5'-oligoadenylate synthetase caused by deoxyoformycin in hairy cell leukaemia. Brit J Haematol 80(2):194, 1992

121. Gasche C, Reinisch W, Schwarzmeier JD: Evidence of colony suppressor activity and deficiency of hematopoietic growth factors in hairy cell leukemia. Hematol Oncol 11(2):97, 1993

122. Gastl G, Werter M, De-Pauw B, Nerl C, Aulitzky W, von-Luttichau I, Tilg H, Thaler J, Lang A, Abbrederis K, et al.: Comparison of clinical efficacy and toxicity of conventional and optimum biological response modifying doses of interferon alpha-2C in the treatment of hairy cell leukemia: a retrospective analysis of 39 patients. Leukemia 3(6):453, 1989

123. Gastl G, Aulitzky W, Tilg H, Thaler J, Berger M, Huber C: Minimal interferon-alpha doses for hairy cell leukemia [letter; comment]. Blood 75(3):812, 1990

124. Gazitt Y, Leizerowitz R, Polliack A: Induction of plasmacytoid and hairy cell features by phorbol esters (TPA) in B-lymphoma cells: attempted correlation with disease activity. Hematol Oncol 6(4):307, 1988

125. Genot E, Leprince C, Richard Y, Petit-Koskas E, Falcoff E, Galanaud P, Sigaux F, Kolb JP: Expression of the B8.7 antigen on hairy cells and relation with the LMW-BCGF response. Leukemia 3(5):367, 1989

126. Genot E, Sarfati M, Sigaux F, Petit-Koskas E, Billard C, Mathiot C, Falcoff E, Delespesse G, Kolb JP: Effect of interferon-alpha on the expression and release of the CD23 molecule in hairy cell leukemia. Blood 74(7):2455, 1989

127. Genot E, Valentine MA, Degos L, Sigaux F, Kolb JP: Hyperphosphorylation of CD20 in hairy cells. Alteration by low molecular weight B cell growth factor and IFN-alpha. J Immunol 146(3):870, 1991

128. Genot E, Bismuth G, Degos L, Sigaux F, Wietzerbin J: Interferon-alpha downregulates the abnormal intracytoplasmic free calcium concentration of tumor cells in hairy cell leukemia. Blood 80(8):2060, 1992

129. Genot EM, Meier KE, Licciardi KA, Ahn NG, Uittenbogaart CH, Wietzerbin J, Clark EA, Valentine MA: Phosphorylation of CD20 in cells from a hairy cell leukemia cell line. Evidence for involvement of calcium/calmodulin-dependent protein kinase II. J Immunol 151(1):71, 1993

130. Genot E, Wietzerbin J: Investigating hairy cell leukemia dysregulations. Looking for interferon alpha site of action on hairy cells. Leuk Lymphoma 14 (suppl 1):23, 1994

131. Giardina SL, Young HA, Faltynek CR, Jaffe ES, Clark JW, Steis RG, Urba WJ, Mathieson BJ, Gralnick H, Lawrence J, et al.: Rearrangement of both immunoglobulin and T-cell receptor genes in a prolymphocytic variant of hairy cell leukemia patient resistant to interferon-alpha. Blood 72(5):1708, 1988 (published erratum appears in Blood 73(2):624, 1989)

132. Glaspy JA, Baldwin GC, Robertson PA, Souza L, Vincent M, Ambersley J, Golde DW: Therapy for neutropenia in hairy cell leukemia with recombinant human granulocyte colony-stimulating factor. Ann Intern Med 109(10):789, 1988

133. Glaspy JA, Marcus SG, Ambersley J, Golde DW: Recombinant beta-serine-interferon in hairy cell leukemia compared prospectively with results with recombinant alpha-interferon. Cancer 64(2):409, 1989

134. Glaspy JA, Souza L, Scates S, Narachi M, Blatt L, Ambersley J, Golde DW: Treatment of hairy cell leukemia with granulocyte colony-stimulating factor and recombinant consensus interferon or recombinant interferon-alpha-2b. J Immunother 11(3):198, 1992

135. Golomb HM, Catovsky D, Golde DW: Hairy cell leukemia. Ann Intern Mede 89:677, 1978

136. Golomb HM, Mintz U, Vardiman J, Wilson C, Rosner MC: Surface immunoglobulin, lectin-induced cap formation and phagocytic function in five patients with the leukemic phase of hairy cell leukemia. Cancer 46:50, 1980

137. Golomb HM: Progress report on chlorambucil therapy in postsplenectomy patients with progressive hairy cell leukemia. Blood 57:464, 1981

138. Golomb HM, Vardiman JW: Response to splenectomy in 65 patients with hairy cell leukemia: an evaluation of spleen weight and bone marrow involvement. Blood 61:349, 1983

139. Golomb HM, Fefer A, Golde DW, Ozer H, Portlock C, Silber R, Rappeport J, Ratain MJ, Thompson J, Bonnem E, et al.: Report of a multi-institutional study of 193 patients with hairy cell leukemia treated with interferon-alfa2b. Semin Oncol 15(5) (suppl 5):7, 1988

140. Golomb HM, Ratain MJ, Fefer A, Thompson J, Golde DW, Ozer H, Portlock C, Silber R, Rappeport J, Bonnem E, et al.: Randomized study of the duration of treatment with interferon alfa-2B in patients with hairy cell leukemia. J Natl Cancer Inst 80(5):369, 1988

141. Golomb HM, Ratain MJ, Mick R, Daly K: Interferon treatment for hairy cell leukemia: an update on a cohort of 69 patients treated from 1983–1986. Leukemia 6(11):1177, 1992
142. Gooi J, Burns GF, Cawley JC: Hairy-cell leukaemia: an immunoperoxidase study of paraffin-embedded tissues. J Clin Pathol 32:1244, 1979
143. Gordon J, Smith JL: Free immunoglobulin light cahin synthesis by neoplastic cells in leukaemic reticuloendotheliosis. Clin Exp Immunol 31:244, 1978
144. Gramatovici M, Bennett JM, Hiscock JG, Grewal KS: Three cases of familial hairy cell leukemia. Am J Hematol 42(4):337, 1993
145. Gressler VH, Weinkauff RE, Franklin WA, Golomb HM: Modulation of the expression of major histocompatibility antigens on splenic hairy cells – differential effect upon *in vitro* treatment with alpha-2b-interferon, gamma-interferon, and interleukin-2. Blood 72(3):1048, 1988
146. Gressler VH, Weinkauff RE, Franklin WA, Golomb HM: Is there a direct differentiation-inducing effect of human recombinant interferon on hairy cell leukemia *in vitro*? Cancer 64(2):374, 1989
147. Griffiths SD, Cawley JC: Alpha-interferon and lymphokine-activated killer cells in hairy cell leukemia. Leukemia 2(6):377, 1988
148. Griffiths SD, Cawley JC: The effect of cytokines, including IL-1, IL-4, and IL-6, in hairy cell proliferation/differentiation. Leukemia 4(5):337, 1990
149. Griffiths SD, Cawley JC: Monocyte/macrophages stimulate hairy cell proliferation. Leuk Lymphoma 4:325, 1991
150. Guerin JM, Meyer P, Habib Y: Listeria-monocytogenes infection and hairy-cell leukemia. Am J Med 83(1):188, 1987
151. Guttermann JU: Cytokine therapeutics: lessons from interferon alpha. Proc Natl Acad Sci USA 91:1198, 1994
152. Habermann TM, Andersen JW, Cassileth PA, Bennett JM, Oken MM: Sequential administration of recombinant interferon alpha and deoxycoformycin in the treatment of hairy cell leukaemia. Brit J Haematol 80(4):466, 1992
153. Haglund U, Juliusson G, Stellan B, Gahrton G: Hairy cell leukemia is characterized by clonal chromosome abnormalities clustered to specific regions. Blood 83(9):2637, 1994
154. Hakimian D, Tallman MS, Kiley C, Peterson L: Detection of minimal residual disease by immunostaining of bone marrow biopsies after 2-chlorodeoxyadenosine for hairy cell leukemia. Blood 82(6):1798, 1993
155. Hamilton-Dutoit SJ, Pallesen G: A survey of Epstein–Barr virus gene expression in sporadic non-Hodgkin's lymphomas. Detection of Epstein–Barr virus in a subset of peripheral T-cell lymphomas. Am J Pathol 140(6):1315, 1992
156. Han T, Sadamori N, Block AM, Xiao H, Henderson ES, Emrich L, Sandberg AA: Cytogenetic studies in chronic lymphocytic leukemia, prolymphocytic leukemia and hairy cell leukemia: a progress report. Nouv Rev Fr Hematol 30(5/6):393, 1988
157. Hanson CA, Ward PC, Schnitzer B: A multilobular variant of hairy cell leukemia with morphologic similarities to T-cell lymphoma. Am J Surg Pathol 13(8):671, 1989
158. Hanson CA, Gribbin TE, Schnitzer B, Schlegelmilch JA, Mitchell BS, Stoolman LM: CD11c (LEU-M5) expression characterizes a B-cell chronic lymphoproliferative disorder with features of both chronic lymphocytic leukemia and hairy cell leukemia [see comments]. Blood 76(11):2360, 1990
159. Hansen DA, Robbins BA, Bylund DJ, Piro LD, Saven A, Ellison DJ: Identification of monoclonal immunoglobulins and quantitative immunoglobulin abnormalities in hairy cell leukemia and chronic lymphocytic leukemia. Am J Clin Pathol 102(5):580, 1994
160. Harvey WH, Harb OS, Kosak ST, Sheaffer JC, Lowe LR, Heerema NA: Interferon-alpha-2b downregulation of oncogenes H-ras, c-raf-2, c-kit, c-myc, c-myb and c-fos in ESKOL, a hairy cell leukemic line, results in temporal perturbation of signal transduction cascade. Leuk Res 18(8):577, 1994
161. Hassan IB, Lantz M, Sundstrom C: Effect of alpha-IFN on cytokine-induced antigen expression and secretion of TNF, LT and IgM in HCL. Leuk Res 15(10):903, 1991
162. Hasselbalch H, Lisse I, Berild D, Videbaek A: Spongy lymphoid myelofibrosis as a predictor of hairy-cell leukemia or a variant of hairy-cell leukemia without hairy-cells. Scand J Haematol 32(2):135, 1984
163. Hasselbalch H, Braide I, Lisse I, Rockert LL, Swolin B, Carneskog J, Hagberg H, Hippe E, Jensen MK, Lundin P, *et al.*: Recombinant interferon-alpha-2b treatment of hairy-cell leukaemia: experience with a low-dose schedule. Eur J Haematol 41(5):438, 1988

164. Heilig B, Mapara M, Brockhaus M, Krauth K, Dorken B: Two types of TNF receptors are expressed on human normal and malignant B lymphocytes. Clin Immunol Immunopathol 61(2) (part 1):260, 1991
165. Heimann PS, Vardiman JW, Stock W, Platanias LC, Golomb HM: CD5+, CD11c+, CD20+ hairy cell leukemia [letter; comment]. Blood 77(7):1617, 1991
166. Herold CJ, Wittich GR, Schwarzinger I, Haller J, Chott A, Mostbeck G, Hajek PC: Skeletal involvement in hairy cell leukemia. Skeletal Radiol 17(3):171, 1988
167. Heslop HE, Bianchi AC, Cordingley FT, Turner M, Chandima W, De-Mel CP, Hoffbrand AV, Brenner MK: Effects of interferon alpha on autocrine growth factor loops in B lymphoproliferative disorders. J Exp Med 172(6):1729, 1990
168. Heslop HE, Brenner MK, Ganeshaguru K, Hoffbrand AV: Possible mechanism of action of interferon alpha in chronic B-cell malignancies. Brit J Haematol 79 (suppl 1):14, 1991
169. Heslop HE, Hoffbrand AV, Brenner MK: TNF and chronic B lymphoproliferative disorders [letter]. Leukemia 7(9):1476, 1993
170. Higuchi M, Aggarwal BB: Differential roles of the two types of TNF receptor in TNF induced cytotoxicity, DNA fragmentation and differentiation b. J Immunol 152:4017, 1994
171. Hirota Y, Yoshioka A, Tanaka S, Wantanbe K, Otani T: Imbalance of deoxyucleotide triphosphates. DNA double strand breaks and cell death caused by 2-chloroeoxyadenosine in mouse FM3A cells. Cancer Res 49:915, 1989
172. Hjelle B, Chaney R: Sequence variation of functional HTLV-II tax alleles among isolates from an endemic population: lack of evidence for oncogenic determinant in tax. J Med Virol 36(2):136, 1992
173. Ho AD, Ganeshaguru K, Knauf WU, Dietz G, Trede I, Hunstein W, Hoffbrand AV: Clinical response to deoxycoformycin in chronic lymphoid neoplasms and biochemical changes in circulating malignant cells in vivo. Blood 72(6):1884, 1988
174. Ho AD, Ganeshaguru K, Knauf W, Dietz G, Trede I, Hoffbrand AV, Hunstein W: Enzyme activities of leukemic cells and biochemical changes induced by deoxycoformycin in vitro – lack of correlation with clinical response. Leuk Res 13(4):269, 1989
175. Ho AD, Thaler J, Mandelli F, Lauria F, Zittoun R, Willemze R, McVie G, Marmont AM, Prummer O, Stryckmans P, et al.: Response to pentostatin in hairy-cell leukemia refractory to interferon-alpha. The European Organization for Research and Treatment of Cancer Leukemia Cooperative Group. J Clin Oncol 7(10):1533, 1989
176. Ho AD, Klotzbucher A, Gross A, Dietz G, Mestan J, Jakobsen H, Hunstein W: Induction of intracellular and plasma 2',5'-oligoadenylate synthetase by pentostatin. Leukemia 6(3):209, 1992
177. Huang D, Reittie JE, Stephens S, Hoffbrand AV, Brenner MK: Effects of anti-TNF monoclonal antibody infusion in patients with hairy cell leukaemia. Brit J Haematol 81(2):231, 1992
178. Fifth International Workshop on Human Differentiation Antigens.: Leukocyte Typing V. White Cell Differentiation Antigens. Oxford, Oxford University Press, 1995
179. Isaacson PG, Matutes E, Burke M, Catovsky D: The histopathology of splenic lymphoma with villous lymphocytes. Blood 84(11):3828, 1994
180. Jabbar SA, Hoffbrand AV, Gitendra-Wickremasinghe R: Regulation of transcription factors NF kappa B and AP-1 following tumour necrosis factor-alpha treatment of cells from chronic B cell leukaemia patients. Brit J Haematol 86(3):496, 1994
181. Jacobs RH, Vokes EE, Golomb HM: Second malignancies in hairy cell leukemia. Cancer 56:1462, 1985
182. Jaiyesimi IA, Kantarjian HM, Estey EH: Advances in therapy for hairy cell leukemia. A review. Cancer 72(1):5, 1993
183. Janckila AJ, Li CY, Lam KW, Yam LT: The cytochemistry of tartrate-resistant acid phosphatase. Technical considerations. Am J Clin Pathol 70:45, 1978
184. Janckila AJ, Gentile PS, Yam LT: Hemopoietic inhibition in hairy cell leukemia. Am J Hematol 38(1):30, 1991
185. Janckila AJ, Latham MD, Lam KW, Chow KC, Li CY, Yam LT: Heterogeneity of hairy cell tartrate-resistant acid phosphatase. Clin Biochem 25(6):437, 1992
186. Janckila AJ, Woodford TA, Lam KW, Li CY, Yam LT: Protein-tyrosine phosphatase activity of hairy cell tartrate-resistant acid phosphatase. Leukemia 6(3):199, 1992
187. Janckila AJ, Cardwell EM, Yam LT, Li CY: Hairy cell identification by immunoytochemistry of tartrate resistant acid phosphatase. Blood 85:2839, 1995
188. Jansen J, Hermans J, Remme J, den Ottolander GJ, Lopes Cardoza P: Hairy cell leukaemia. Clinical features and effect of splenectomy. Scand J Haematol 21:60, 1978

189. Jansen J, Hermans J: Splenectomy in hairy cell leukemia: a retrospective multicenter analysis. Cancer 47:2066, 1981
190. Jansen J, Hermans J: Clinical staging system for hairy-cell leukemia. Blood 60:571, 1982
191. Jansen J, Schuit HRE, Meijer JLM, van Nieuwkoop JA, Hijmans W: Cell markers in hairy cell leukemia studied in cells from 51 patients. Blood 59:52, 1982
192. Jansen J, Bolhuis RLH, Vanieuwkoop JA, Schuit HRE, Kroese WFS: Paraproteinemia plus osteolytic lesions in typical hairy-cell leukemia. Brit J Haematol 54(4):531, 1983
193. Jansen JH, van-der-Harst D, Wientjens GJ, Kooy-Winkelaar YM, Brand A, Willemze R, Kluin-Nelemans HC: Induction of CD11a/leukocyte function antigen-1 and CD54/intercellular adhesion molecule-1 on hairy cell leukemia cells is accompanied by enhanced susceptibility to T-cell but not lymphokine-activated killer-cell cytotoxicity [see comments]. Blood 80(2):478, 1992
194. Jansen JH, Wientjens GJ, Fibbe WE, Ralph P, Van-Damme J, den-Ottolander GJ, Willemze R, Kluin-Nelemans JC: Serum monocyte colony-stimulating factor, erythropoietin and interleukin-6 in relation to pancytopenia in hairy cell leukemia. Leukemia 6(7):735, 1992
195. Jansen JH, Wientjens GJ, Willemze R, Kluin-Nelemans JC: Production of tumor necrosis factor-alpha by normal and malignant B lymphocytes in response to interferon-alpha, interferon-gamma and interleukin-4 [see comments]. Leukemia 6(2):116, 1992
196. Johansson T, Bostrom H, Sjodahl R, Ihse I: Splenectomy for haematological diseases. Acta Chir Scand 156(1):83, 1990
197. Juliusson G, Liliemark J: Rapid recovery from cytopenia in hairy cell leukemia after treatment with 2-chloro-2'-deoxyadenosine (CdA): relation to opportunistic infections. Blood 79(4):888, 1992
198. Juliusson G, Gahrton G: Cytogenetics in CLL and related disorders, in Rozman C (ed): Bailliere's Clinical Haematology (vol 6:4). London, Bailliere Tindall, 1993, p 821
199. Juliusson G, Lenkei R, Liliemark J: Flow cytometry of blood and bone marrow cells from patients with hairy cell leukemia: phenotype of hairy cells and lymphocyte subsets after treatment with 2-chlorodeoxyadenosine. Blood 83(12):3672, 1994
200. Kalyanaraman VS, Sarngadharan MG, Robertguroff M, Miyoshi I, Blayney D, Golde D, Gallo RC: A new subtype of human t-cell leukemia-virus (htlv-II) associated with a t-cell variant of hairy-cell leukemia. Science 218(4572):571, 1982
201. Kampmeier P, Spielberger R, Dickstein J, Mick R, Golomb H, Vardiman JW: Increased incidence of second neoplasms in patients treated with interferon alpha 2b for hairy cell leukemia: a clinicopathologic assessment. Blood 83(10):2931, 1994
202. Kantarjian HM, Schachner J, Keating MJ: Fludarabine therapy in hairy cell leukemia. Cancer 67(5):1291, 1991
203. Karray S, Leprince C, Merle-Beral H, Debre P, Richard Y, Galanaud P: B8.7 antigen expression on B-CLL cells and its relationship to the LMW-BCGF responsiveness. Leuk Res 14(9):809, 1990
204. Katayama I, Li CY, Yam LT: Histochemical study of acid phosphatase isoenzyme in leukemic reticuloendotheliosis. Cancer 29:157, 1972
205. Katayama I, Finkel HE: Leukemic reticuiloendotheliosis. A clinicopathologic study with review of literature. Am J Med 57:115, 1974
206. Katayama I, Schneider GB: Further ultrastructural characterisation of hairy cells of leukemic reticuloendotheliosis. Am J Pathol 86:163, 1977
207. Katayama I, Shimizu M: Hairy-cell leukemia in Japan. Lab Invest 50(1), 1984
208. Katayama I, Hirashima K, Maruyama K, Hoshino S, Abe T, Furusawa S, Iguchi Y: Hairy-cell leukemia in Japanese patients – a study with monoclonal antibodies. Leukemia 1(4):301, 1987
209. Kayano H, Dyer MJ, Zani VJ, Laffan MA, Matutes E, Asou N, Katayama I, Catovsky D: Aberrant rearrangements within the immunoglobulin heavy chain locus in hairy cell leukemia. Leuk Lymphoma 14 (suppl 1):41, 1994
210. Kloke O, May D, Wandl U, Niederle N: [The dose of alpha interferon in induction and maintainance therapy of hairy cell leukemia]. Onkologie 11 (suppl 2):41, 1988
211. Kluin-Nelemans HC, Krouwels MM, Jansen JH, Dijkstra K, van-Tol MJ, den-Ottolander GJ, Dreef EJ, Kluin PM: Hairy cell leukemia preferentially expresses the IgG3-subclass. Blood 75(4):972, 1990
212. Kluin-Nelemans HC, Beverstock GC, Mollevanger P, Wessels HW, Hoogendoorn E, Willemze R, Falkenburg JH: Proliferation and cytogenetic analysis of hairy cell leukemia upon stimulation via the CD40 antigen. Blood 84(9):3134, 1994
213. Kluin-Nelemans JC, Kester MG, Oving I, Cluitmans FH, Willemze R, Falkenburg JH:

Abnormally activated T lymphocytes in the spleen of patients with hairy-cell leukemia. Leukemia 8(12):2095, 1994

214. Knapp W, Dorken B, Gilks WR, Rieber EP, Schmidt RE, Stein H, von dem Borne AEGK, eds: Leukocyte Typing IV. White Cell Differentiation Antigens. Oxford, Oxford University Press, 1989

215. Knecht H, Rhyner K, Streuli RA: Toxoplasmosis in hairy-cell leukemia. Brit J Haematol 62(1):65, 1986

216. Komminoth A, Dufour P, Bergerat JP, Wiesel ML, Falkenrodt A, Oberling F: Hairy cell leukemia and factor VIII inhibitor: a case report. Nouv Rev Fr Hematol 34(3):269, 1992

217. Korsmeyer SJ, Greene WC, Cossman J: Rearrangement and expression of immunoglobulin genes and expression of Tac antigen in hairy cell leukemia. Proc Natl Acad Sci USA 80:4522, 1983

218. Krause JR, Strodes C, Lee RE: Use of the bone marrow imprint in the diagnosis of leukemic reticuloendotheliosis. Am J Clin Pathol 68:368, 1977

219. Kraut EH, Bouroncle BA, Grever MR: Pentostatin in the treatment of advanced hairy cell leukemia. J Clin Oncol 7(2):168, 1989

220. Kraut EH, Chun HG: Fludarabine phosphate in refractory hairy cell leukemia. Am J Hematol 37(1):59, 1991

221. Kuratsune H, Owada MK, Tokumine Y, Tagawa S, Nojima J, Shibano M, Nishimori Y, Morita T, Machii T, Kitani T: Association of protein tyrosine phosphorylation with B cell differentiation induced by 12-O-tetradecanoylphorbol-13-acetate (TPA). Leukemia 4(10):700, 1990

222. Lahat N, Aghai E, Merchav S, Kinarty A, Sobel E, Froom P: Concomitant effect of 2'-deoxycoformycin on natural killer cell activity and tumour cell sensitivity to lysis in hairy cell leukaemia – discordant effects of alpha interferon. Scand J Immunol 32(2):205, 1990

223. Laughlin M, Islam A, Barcos M, Meade P, Ozer H, Gavigan M, Henderson E, Han T: Effect of alpha-interferon therapy on bone marrow fibrosis in hairy cell leukemia. Blood 72(3):936, 1988

224. Lauria F, Bagnara GP, Catani L, Gaggioli L, Guarini A, Raspadori D, Foa R, Bellone G, Buzzi M, Gugliotta L, et al.: The inhibitory effect of serum from hairy-cell leukaemia patients on normal progenitor cells may disappear following prolonged treatment with alpha-interferon. Brit J Haematol 72(4):497, 1989

225. Lauria F, Raspadori D, Foa R, Zinzani PL, Buzzi M, Gugliotta L, Macchi S, Tura S: Reduced hematologic response to alpha-interferon therapy in patients with hairy cell leukemia showing a peculiar immunologic phenotype. Cancer 65(10):2233, 1990

226. Lauria F, Raspadori D, Benfenati D, Rondelli D, Pallotti A, Tura S: Biological markers and minimal residual disease in hairy cell leukemia. Leukemia 6 (suppl 4):149, 1992

227. Lauria F, Benfenati D, Raspadori D, Rondelli D, Ventura MA, Pileri S, Sabattini E, Poggi S, Benni M, Tura S: Retreatment with 2-CdA of progressed HCL patients. Leuk Lymphoma 14 (suppl 1):143, 1994

228. Lebezu M, Pinaudeau Y, Poirier J, Dreyfus B: Involvement of the nervous system in hairy-cell leukemia. Arch Neurol 42(9):839, 1985

229. Lehn P, Sigaux F, Grausz D, Loiseau P, Castaigne S, Degos L, Flandarin G, Dautry F: C-myc and C-fos expression during interferon alpha therapy for hairy cell leukaemia. Blood 68:967, 1986

230. Lembersky BC, Ratain MJ, Golomb HM: Skeletal complications in hairy cell leukemia: diagnosis and therapy. J Clin Oncol 6(8):1280, 1988

231. Levine MA, Toback AC: Enhancement of granulopoiesis by lithium carbonate in a patient with hairy-cell leukemia. Am J Med 82:146, 1987

232. Lewis SM, Catovsky D, Hows JM, Ardalan B: Splenic red cell pooling in hairy cell leukaemia. Brit J Haematol 35:351, 1977

233. Lewis JP, Tanke HJ, Raap AK, Kibbelaar RE, Kluin PM, Kluin-Nelemans HC: Hairy cell leukemia: an interphase cytogenetic study. Leukemia 7(9):1334, 1993

234. Li CY, Yam LT, Lam KW: Studies of acid phospahatase isoenzymes in human leukocytes. Demonstration of isoenzyme cell specificity. J Histochem Cytochem 18:901, 1970

235. Liberati AM, Fizzotti M, Di-Clemente F, Senatore M, Berruto P, Falini B, Martelli MF, Grignani F: Response to intermediate and standard doses of IFN-beta in hairy-cell leukaemia. Leuk Res 14(9):779, 1990

236. Liberati AM, Horisberger M, Schippa M, Di-Clemente F, Fizzotti M, Filippo S, Proietti MG, Arzano S, Berruto P, Palmisano L, et al.: Biochemical and immunological responses of hairy cell leukemia patients to interferon beta. Cancer Immunol Immunother 34(2):115, 1991

237. Liberati AM, Schippa M, Portuesi MG, Grazia-Proietti M, De-Angelis V, Ferrajoli A, Cinieri S,

Di-Clemente F, Palmisano L, Berruto P: IFN-beta induced biochemical and immunological modifications in hairy cell leukemia patients. Haematologica 76(5):375, 1991

238. Lindemann A, Ludwig WD, Oster W, Mertelsmann R, Herrmann F: High-level secretion of tumor necrosis factor-alpha contributes to hematopoietic failure in hairy cell leukemia [see comments]. Blood 73(4):880, 1989

239. Lindemann A, Herrmann F, Mertelsmann R, Gamm H, Rumpelt HJ: Splenic hematopoiesis following GM-CSF therapy in a patient with hairy cell leukemia [letter]. Leukemia 4(8):606, 1990

240. Lion T, Razvi N, Golomb HM, Brownstein RH: B-lymphocytic hairy cells contain no HTLV-II DNA sequences. Blood 72(4):1428, 1988

241. Lisse I, Hasselbalch H, Junker P: Bone marrow stroma in idiopathic myelofibrosis and other haematological diseases. Apmis 99:171, 1991

242. Loewy AG: The cytoplasmic matrix and the conversion of chemical energy into work, in Loewy AG, Siekevtz P, Menninger JR, Gallant JAN (eds): Cell Structure And Function. Philadelphia, Saunders, 1991

243. Lorber C, Willfort A, Ohler L, Jager U, Schwarzinger I, Lechner K, Geissler K: Granulocyte colony-stimulating factor (rh G-CSF) as an adjunct to interferon alpha therapy of neutropenic patients with hairy cell leukemia. Ann Hematol 67(1):13, 1993

244. Lower EE, Franco RS, Martelo OJ: Increased tyrosine protein kinase activity in hairy cell and monocytic leukemias. Am J Med Sci 303(6):387, 1992

245. Lui YJ, Zhang J, Lane PJL, Chan EYT, MacLennan ICM: Sites of specific B cell activation in primary and secondary responses to T cell-dependent and independent antigens. Eur J Immunol 1991:2951, 1991

246. Lynch SA, Brugge JS, Fromowitz F, Glantz L, Wang P, Caruso R, Viola MV: Increased expression of the src proto-oncogene in hairy cell leukemia and a subgroup of B-cell lymphomas. Leukemia 7(9):1416, 1993

247. Machii T, Tokumine Y, Inoue R, Kitani T: A unique variant of hairy cell leukemia in Japan. Jpn J Med 29(4):379, 1990

248. MacLennan ICM: Germinal Centers. Annu Rev Immunol 12:117, 1994

249. Maher DW, Pike BL, Boyd AW: The response of human B cells to interleukin 4 is determined by their stage of activation and differentiation. Scand J Immunol 32(6):631, 1990

250. Manconi R, Poletti A, Volpe R, Sulfaro S, Carbone A: Dendritic reticulum cell pattern as a microenvironmental indicator for a distinct origin of lymphoma of follicular mantle cells. Brit J Haematol 68(2):213, 1988

251. Mantovani G, Astara G, Curreli L, Lai P, Turnu E, Locci F, Lantini MS, Cossu M, Riva A, Del-Giacco GS: Ultrastructural, immunologic and clinical follow-up of five patients with HCL treated with interferon (IFN) for more than three years. Haematologica 77(4):326, 1992

252. Marie JP, Degos L, Flandrin G: Hairy cell leukaemia and tuberculosis. N Engl J Med 297:1354, 1977

253. Marinone GM, Roncoli B: Selective myeloid aplasia: a long-lasting presentation of an unusual hairy cell leukemia variant? Haematologica 78(4):239, 1993

254. Martin JM, Boras VF, Houwen B, Francovich N: Hairy cell leukemia and anti-leukocyte common antigen. Am J Clin Pathol 90(4):412, 1988

255. Masuda M, Takanashi M, Motoji T, Oshimi K, Mizoguchi H: Effect of recombinant interferons on hairy cell leukemia progenitors. Int J Cell Cloning 7(2):120, 1989

256. Matsumoto SS, Yu AL, Yu J: Morphological changes in leukemic lymphoblasts and normal lymphocytes treated with deoxyadenosine plus deoxycoformycin. Cancer Invest 3:325, 1985

257. Matutes E, Morilla R, Owusu-Ankomah K, Houliham A, Meeus P, Catovsky D: The immunophenotype of hairy cell leukemia (HCL). Proposal for a scoring system to distinguish HCL from B-cell disorders with hairy or villous lymphocytes. Leuk Lymphoma 14 (suppl 1):57, 1994

258. McKinney PA, Cartwright RA, Pearlman B: Hairy cell leukemia and occupational exposures [letter]. Brit J Haematol 68(1):142, 1988

259. Mehta AB, Catovsky D, O'Brien CJ, Lott M, Bowley N, Hemmingway A: Massive retroperitoneal lymphadenopathy as a terminal event in hairy-cell leukemia. Clin Lab Haematol 5(3):259, 1983

260. Melo JV, Robinson DSF, Gregory C, Catovsky D: Splenic b-cell lymphoma with villous lymphocytes in the peripheral-blood – a disorder distinct from hairy-cell leukemia. Leukemia 1(4):294, 1987

261. Mercieca J, Matutes E, Moskovic E, MacLennan K, Matthey F, Costello C, Behrens J, Basu S,

Roath S, Fairhead S, et al.: Massive abdominal lymphadenopathy in hairy cell leukaemia: a report of 12 cases. Brit J Haematol 82(3):547, 1992

262. Mercieca J, Puga M, Matutes E, Moskovic E, Salim S, Catovsky D: Incidence and significance of abdominal lymphadenopathy in hairy cell leukaemia. Leuk Lymphoma 14 (suppl 1):79, 1994

263. Micklem KJ, Dong Y, Willis A, Pulford KA, Visser L, Durkop H, Poppema S, Stein H, Mason DY: HML-1 antigen on mucosa-associated T cells, activated cells, and hairy leukemic cells is a new integrin containing the beta 7 subunit. Am J Pathol 139(6):1297, 1991

264. Miller ML, Fishleder AJ, Tubbs RR: The expression of CD22 (Leu 14) and CD11c (LeuM5) in chronic lymphoproliferative disorders using two-color flow cytometric analysis. Am J Clin Pathol 96(1):100, 1991

265. Moller P, Mielke B, Moldenhauer G: Monoclonal antibody HML-1, a marker for intraepithelial T cells and lymphomas derived thereof, also recognizes hairy cell leukemia and some B-cell lymphomas. Am J Pathol 136(3):509, 1990

266. Mongini P, Seremetis S, Blessinger C, Rudich S, Winchester R, Brunda M: Diversity in inhibitory effects of IFN-gamma and IFN-alpha A on the induced DNA synthesis of a hairy cell leukemia B lymphocyte clone reflects the nature of the activating ligand. Blood 72(5):1553, 1988

267. Moormeier JA, Ratain MJ, Westbrook CA, Vardiman JW, Daly KM, Golomb HM: Low-dose interferon alfa-2b in the treatment of hairy cell leukemia. J Natl Cancer Inst 81(15):1172, 1989

268. Morroni M, Ripa G, Bolognesi G, Leoni P, Cinti S: Ultrastructural modifications in one case of hairy cell leukemia during alpha-interferon therapy. Tumori 78(3):190, 1992

269. Naeim F, Smith GS: Leukemic reticuloendotheliosis. Cancer 34:1813, 1974

270. Nakamura Y, Machii T, Tokumine Y: Hairy cells from hairy cell leukemia patients presenting with pronounced polyclonal hypergammaglobulinaemia secrete a factor enhancing IgG synthesis. Clin Immunol Immunopathol 66:212, 1993

271. Nanba K, Jaffe ES, Soban EJ, Braylan RC, Berard CW: Hairy cell leukemia. Enzyme histochemical characterisation, with special reference to splenic stromal changes. Cancer 39:2323, 1977

272. Nanba K, Soban EJ, Bowling MC, Berad CW: Splenic pseudosinuses and hepatic angiomatous lesions. Distinctive features of hairy cell leukemia. Am J Clin Pathol 67:415, 1977

273. Narni F, Mariano MT, Moretti L, Colo A, Montagnani G, Grantini M, Donelli A, Torelli U: Atypical pattern of light chain gene rearrangement in hairy cell leukemia. Hematol Pathol 5(1):11, 1991

274. Neiman RS, Sullivan AL, Jaffe R: Malignant lymphoma simulating leukemic reticulo-ndotheliosis: a clinico-pathologic study of 10 cases. Cancer 43:329, 1979

275. Ng JP, Hogg RB, Cumming RLC, McCallion J, Catovsky D: Primary splenic hairy-cell leukemia – a case-report and review of the literature. Eur J Haematol 39(4):349, 1987

276. Niederle N, Doberauer C, Kloke O, Hoffken K, Schmidt CG: Effectiveness of gamma interferon and alpha interferon in hairy cell leukemia. Klin Wochenschr 65:706, 1987

277. Nielsen B, Hokland M, Justesen J, Hasselbalch H, Ellegaard J, Hokland P: Immunological recovery and dose evaluation in IFN-alpha treatment of hairy cell leukemia: analysis of leukocyte differentiation antigens, NK and 2',5'-oligoadenylate synthetase activity. Eur J Haematol 42(1):50, 1989

278. Nielsen B, Hokland P, Ellegaard J, Hasselbalch H, Hokland M: Whole blood assay for NK activity in splenectomized and non-splenectomized hairy cell leukemia patients during IFN-alpha-2b treatment. Leuk Res 13(6):451, 1989

279. Nielsen B, Braide I: Three years' continuous low-dose interferon-alpha treatment of hairy-cell leukaemia: evaluation of response and maintenance dose. Eur J Haematol 49(4):174, 1992

280. Nielsen B, Braide I, Hasselbalch H: Evidence for an association between hairy cell leukemia and renal cell and colorectal carcinoma. Cancer 70(8):2087, 1992

281. Nobes CD, Hall A: Rho, Rac, and Cdc42 GTPases regulate the assembly of multiolecular focal complexes associated with actin stress fibres, lamellipodia, and filopodia. Cell 81:53, 1995

282. Ohsawa M, Kanno H, Machii T, Aozasa K: Immunoreactivity of neoplastic and non-neoplastic monocytoid B lymphocytes for DBA.44 and other antibodies. J Clin Pathol 47(10):928, 1994

283. Oleske D, Golomb HM, Farber MD, Levy PS: A case-control inquiry into the etiology of hairy-cell leukemia. Am J Epidemiol 121(5):675, 1985

284. Ozes ON, Klein SB, Reiter Z, Taylor MW: An interferon resistant variant of the hairy-cell leukemic cell line, Eskol: biochemical and immunological characterization. Leuk Res 17(11):983, 1993

285. Palumbo AP, Corradini P, Battaglio S, Omede P, Coda R, Boccadoro M, Pileri A: Dual

rearrangement of immunoglobulin and T-cell receptor gene in a case of T-cell hairy-cell leukemia. Eur J Haematol 46(2):71, 1991

286. Pangalis GA, Boussiotis VA, Kittas C, Panaiotidis PG, Mitsoulis-Mentzikoff C, Loukopoulos D, Fessas P: Hairy cell leukemia: residual splenic disease after successul interferon therapy. Leuk Lymphoma 6:145, 1992

287. Pascali E, Pezzoli A: The clinical spectrum of pure Bence Jones proteinuria. A study of 66 patients. Cancer 62(11):2408, 1988

288. Pellegrini S, Schindler C: Early events in signalling by interferons. TIBS 18:338, 1993

289. Pilarski LM, Masellis-Smith A, Belch AR, Yang B, Savani RC, Turley EA: RHAMM, a receptor for hyaluronan-mediated motility, on normal human lymphocytes, thymocytes and malignant B cells: a mediator in B cell malignancy? Leuk Lymphoma 14(5/6):363, 1994

290. Pileri S, Sabattini E, Poggi S, Merla E, Raspadori D, Benfenati D, Rondelli D, Benni M, Ventura MA, Falini B, et al.: Bone-marrow biopsy in hairy cell leukaemia (HCL) patients. Histological and immunohistological analysis of 46 cases treated with different therapies. Leuk Lymphoma 14 (suppl 1):67, 1994

291. Pilon VA, Davey FR, Gordon GB: Splenic alterations in hairy-cell leukemia. Arch Pathol Lab Med 105(11):577, 1981

292. Pilon VA, Davey FR, Gordon GB, Jones DB: Splenic alterations in hairy-cell leukemia .2. an electron-microscopic study. Cancer 48(7):1617, 1982

293. Piro LD, Carrera CJ, Carson DA, Beutler E: Lasting remissions in hairy-cell leukemia induced by a single infusion of 2-chlorodeoxyadenosine. N Engl J Med 322(16):1117, 1990

294. Piro LD, Ellison DJ, Saven A: The Scripps Clinic experience with 2-chlorodeoxydenosine in the treatment of hairy cell leukemia. Leuk Lymphoma 14 (suppl 1):121, 1994

295. Pittaluga S, Verhoef G, Maes A, Boogaerts MA, De-Wolf-Peeters C: Bone marrow trephines. Findings in patients with hairy cell leukaemia before and after treatment. Histopathology 25(2):129, 1994

296. Platanias LC, Pfeffer LM, Barton KP, Vardiman JW, Golomb HM, Colamonici OR: Expression of the IFN alpha receptor in hairy cell leukaemia. Brit J Haematol 82(3):541, 1992

297. Pope A, Lazarchick J, Hoyer L, Weinstein A: Hairy-cell leukemia and vasculitis. J Rheumatol 7(6):895, 1980

298. Porzsolt F, Demeter J, Heimpel H: Functional criteria for staging and treatment of hairy cell leukemia. Onkologie 14(1):44, 1991

299. Porzsolt F, Schmid M, Staib G, Schrezenmeier H: Paracrine regulation of B-cell growth in hairy cell leukemia. Leuk Lymphoma 14 (suppl 1):13, 1994

300. Posnett DN, Duggan A, McGrath H: Hairy cell leukemia-associated antigen (HC2) is an activation antigen of several hemopoietic cell lineages, inducible on monocytes by IFN-gamma. J Immunol 144(3):929, 1990

301. Pralle H, Bartel A, Boedewadt-Radzun S, Bross K, Bruhn HD, Dorken B, Drees N, Essers U, Fuhr H, Gamm H, et al.: [Alpha interferon in the therapy of hairy-cell leukemia. Results of three prospective multicentre studies in West Germany]. Onkologie 11(1):44, 1988

302. Quesada JR, Itri L, Gutterman JV: Alpha interferon in HCL – a five year followup in one hundred patients. J Interferon Res 7:678, 1987

303. Rai KR: Comparison of pentostatin and alpha interferon in splenectomized patients with active hairy cell leukemia: an intergroup study. Cancer and Leukemia Group B and South-West Oncology Group. Leuk Lymphoma 14 (suppl 1):107, 1994

304. Ratain MJ, Golomb HM, Vardiman JW, Westbrook CA, Barker C, Hooberman A, Bitter MA, Daly K: Relapse after interferon alfa-2b therapy for hairy-cell leukemia: analysis of prognostic variables. J Clin Oncol 6(11):1714, 1988

305. Ratain MJ, Vardiman JW, Barker CM, Golomb HM: Prognostic variables in hairy cell leukemia after splenectomy as initial therapy. Cancer 62(11):2420, 1988

306. Re G, Pileri S, Cau R, Bucchi ML, Casali AM, Cavalli G: Histometry of splenic microvascular architecture in hairy cell leukaemia. Histopathology 13(4):425, 1988

307. Reiter Z, Ozes ON, Blatt LM, Taylor MW: Cytokine and natural killing regulation of growth of a hairy cell leukemia-like cell line: the role of interferon-alpha and interleukin-2. J Immunother 11(1):40, 1992

308. Reiter Z, Taylor MW: Interleukin 2 protects hairy leukemic cells from lymphokine-activated killer cell-mediated cytotoxicity. Cancer Res 53(15):3555, 1993

309. Renshaw BR, Fanslow WC, Armitage RJ, Campbell KA, Liggitt D, Wright B, Davison BL,

Maliszweski CR: Humoural immune responses in CD40 ligand-deficient mice. J Exp Med 180:1889, 1994

310. Richards JM, Mick R, Latta JM, Daly K, Ratain MJ, Vardiman JW, Golomb HM: Serum soluble interleukin-2 receptor is associated with clinical and pathologic disease status in hairy cell leukemia [see comments]. Blood 76(10):1941, 1990

311. Robbins BA, Ellison DJ, Spinosa JC, Carey CA, Lukes RJ, Poppema S, Saven A, Piro LD: Diagnostic application of two-color flow cytometry in 161 cases of hairy cell leukemia. Blood 82(4):1277, 1993

312. Ross SR, McTavish D, Faulds D: Fludarabine. A review of its pharmacological properties and therapeutic potential in malignancy. Drugs 45:737, 1993

313. Rosso R, Neiman RS, Paulli M, Boveri E, Kindl S, Magrini U, Barosi G: Splenic marginal zone cell lymphoma: report of an indolent variant without massive splenomegaly presumably representing an early phase of the disease. Hum Pathol 26(1):39, 1995

314. Ruoslahti E: Control of cell motility and tumour invasion by extracellular matrix interactions. Brit J Cancer 66:239, 1992

315. Sainati L, Matutes E, Mulligan S, de-Oliveira MP, Rani S, Lampert IA, Catovsky D: A variant form of hairy cell leukemia resistant to alpha-interferon: clinical and phenotypic characteristics of 17 patients. Blood 76(1):157, 1990

316. Salvarani C, Capozzoli N, Baricchi R, Macchioni PL, Rossi F, Ghirelli L, Bellelli A, Tumiati B, Portioli I: Autoimmune disease in hairy-cell leukemia: systemic vasculitis and anticardiolipin syndrome [letter]. Clin Exp Rheumatol 7(3):329, 1989

317. Santagati G, Nastasi G, Porta C, Moroni M, Santagati C, Casagranda I, Bobbio-Pallavicini E, Cosimi MF: Low doses of alpha 2B interferon in the treatment of hairy cell leukemia: results of treatment and mean follow-up at 18 months in 13 patients. Pathologica 86(1):66, 1994

318. Saven A, Piro L: Newer purine analogues for the treatment of hairy-cell leukemia. N Engl J Med 330(10):691, 1994

319. Schiller JH, Bittner G, Spriggs DR: Tumor necrosis factor, but not other hematopoietic growth factors, prolongs the survival of hairy cell leukemia cells. Leuk Res 16(4):337, 1992

320. Schlossman SF, Boumsell L, Gilks W, Harlan JM, Kishimoto T, Morimoto C, Ritz J, Shaw S, Silverstein R, Springer T, Tedder TF, Todd RF, eds: Leukocyte Typing V. White Cell Differentiation Antigens (vol I and II). Oxford, Oxford University Press, 1995

321. Schwarting R, Stein H, Wang CY: The monoclonal-antibodies alpha-s-hcl1 and alpha-s-hcl3 allow the diagnosis of hairy-cell leukemia. Blood 65:974, 1985

322. Schweizer CM, van der Valk P, Thijsen SFT, Drager AM, van der Schoot CE, Zevenberg A, Theijsmeijer AP, Langenhuijsen MMAC: Constitutive expression of ELAM and VCAM adhesion molecules in hematopoetic organs. Blood 84 (suppl):929, 1994

323. Semenzato G, Trentin L, Zambello R, Agostini C, Bulian P, Siviero F, Ambrosetti A, Vinante F, Prior M, Chilosi M, et al.: Origin of the soluble interleukin-2 receptor in the serum of patients with hairy cell leukemia. Leukemia 2(12):788, 1988

324. Semenzato G, Trentin L, Zambello R, Agostini C, Chisesi T, Pizzolo G: Hairy cell sensitivity to the lysis in vitro. Role of the anti-CD3 antibody in generating a susceptibility to the lysis. Cancer Immunol Immunother 30(4):254, 1989

325. Seshadri RS, Brown EJ, Zipursky A: Leukemic reticuloendotheliosis. A failure of monocyte production. N Engl J Med 295:181, 1976

326. Seto S, Carrera CJ, Wasson DB: Inhibition of DNA repair by deoxyadenosine in resting human lymphocytes. J Immunol 136:2839, 1986

327. Seymour JF, Kurzrock R, Freireich EJ, Estey EH: 2-Chlorodeoxyadenosine induces durable remissions and prolonged suppression of CD4+ lymphocyte counts in patients with hairy cell leukemia. Blood 83(10):2906, 1994

328. Sheibani K, Sohn K, Burke JS, Winberg CD, Wu AM, Rappaport H: Monocytoid B-cell lymphoma. A novel B-cell neoplasm. Am J Pathol 124:310, 1986

329. Sheibani K, Burke JS, Swartz WG, Nademanee A, Winberg CD: Monocytoid B-cell lymphoma. Clinicopathologic study of 21 cases of a unique type of low-grade lymphoma. Cancer 62:1531, 1988

330. Simonten SC, Basra ML, Barnes DW, Furcht LT: Distribution and immunoocalisation of serum spreading factor in human tissue. Lab Invest 52:63A, 1985

331. Smalley RV, Anderson SA, Tuttle RL, Connors J, Thurmond LM, Huang A, Castle K, Magers C, Whisnant JK: A randomized comparison of two doses of human lymphoblastoid interferon-alpha in hairy cell leukemia. Wellcome HCL Study Group. Blood 78(12):3133, 1991

332. Smalley RV, Connors J, Tuttle RL, Anderson S, Robinson W, Whisnant JK: Splenectomy vs. alpha interferon: a randomized study in patients with previously untreated hairy cell leukemia. Am J Hematol 41(1):13, 1992

333. Smith JW 2d, Longo DL, Urba WJ, Clark JW, Watson T, Beveridge J, Conlon KC, Sznol M, Creekmore SP, Alvord WG, et al.: Prolonged, continuous treatment of hairy cell leukemia patients with recombinant interferon-alpha 2a. Blood 78(7):1664, 1991

334. Snapper CM, Finkelman FD: Immunoglobulin class switching, in Paul WE (ed.): Fundermental Immunology (3rd edn). New York, Raven Press, 1993, p 337

335. Spiegel RJ, Jacobs SL, Treuhaft MW: Anti-interferon antibodies to interferon-alpha 2b: results of comparative assays and clinical perspective. J Interferon Res 9 (suppl 1):S17, 1989

336. Spriggs AI: Hairy cells. Lancet i:427, 1976

337. Springer TA: Adhesion receptors of the immune system. Nature 346:425, 1990

338. Staines A, Cartwright RA: Hairy-cell leukaemia; descriptive epidemiology and a case-control study. Brit J Haematol 85:714, 1993

339. Stang-Voss C, Moebius M: Zur ultrastructure des sogenannten ribosomen-lammellen-komplexes bei haarzell-leukamie. Anat Ges Verh 70:931, 1976

340. Starling GC, Nimmo JC, Hart DN: Hairy cell leukemia cells are relatively NK-insensitive targets. Pathology 20(4):361, 1988

341. Stass SA, Holloway ML, Slease RB, Schumacher HR: Spurious platelet counts in hairy cell leukemia. Am J Clin Pathol 68:530, 1977

342. Steinberg JJ, Suhrland M, Valensi Q: The spleen in the spleen syndrome: the association of splenoma with hematopoietic and neoplastic disease – compendium of cases since 1864. J Surg Oncol 47(3):193, 1991

343. Steinhoff G, Behrend M, Schrader B, Duijvesjin AM, Wongeit K: Expression patterns of leukocyte adhesion ligand molecules on human liver endothelium. Am J Clin Pathol 142:481, 1993

344. Steis RG, Marcon L, Clark J, Urba W, Longo DL, Nelson DL, Maluish AE: Serum soluble IL-2 receptor as a tumor marker in patients with hairy cell leukemia. Blood 71(5):1304, 1988

345. Steis RG, Smith JW 2d, Urba WJ, Clark JW, Itri LM, Evans LM, Schoenberger C, Longo DL: Resistance to recombinant interferon alfa-2a in hairy-cell leukemia associated with neutralizing anti-interferon antibodies. N Engl J Med 318(22):1409, 1988

346. Steis RG, Smith JW 2d, Urba WJ, Venzon DJ, Longo DL, Barney R, Evans LM, Itri LM, Ewel CH: Loss of interferon antibodies during prolonged continuous interferon-alpha 2a therapy in hairy cell leukemia. Blood 77(4):792, 1991

347. Stewart DJ, Keating MJ: Radiation exposure as a possible risk etiologic factor in hairy cell leukaemia. Cancer 46:1577, 1980

348. Stossel P: From signal to pseudopod. J Biol Chem 110:1405, 1989

349. Strickler JG, Schmidt CM, Wick MR: Methods in pathology. Immunophenotype of hairy cell leukemia in paraffin sections. Mod Pathol 3(4):518, 1990

350. Stroup R, Sheibani K: Antigenic phenotypes of hairy cell leukemia and monocytoid B-cell lymphoma: an immunohistochemical evaluation of 66 cases. Hum Pathol 23(2):172, 1992

351. Subramanian VP, Gomez GA, Han T, Kim U, Minowada J, Sandberg A: Coexistence of myeloid metaplasia with myelofibrosis and hairy-cell leukemia. Arch Intern Med 145(1):164, 1985

352. Takahashi K, Umeda S, Shultz LD, Hayashi S, Nishikawa S: Effects of macrophage colony stimulating factor on the development, differentiation and maturation of marginal metallophillic macrophages and marginal zone macrophages in the spleen of osteopetrotic (op) mutant mice lacking functional M-CSF activity. J Leukoc Biol 55:581, 1994

353. Tallman MS, Hakimian D, Dyrda S, Kiley C, Nemcek A, Peterson L: Assessment of complete remission after 2-chlorodeoxyadenosine for hairy cell leukemia: utility of marrow immunostaining and measurement of splenic index. Leuk Lymphoma 14 (suppl 1):133, 1994

354. Tamaki T, Kanakura Y, Kuriu A, Ikeda H, Mitsui H, Yagura H, Matsumura I, Druker B, Griffin JD, Kanayama Y, et al.: Surface immunoglobulin-mediated signal transduction involves rapid phosphorylation and activation of the protooncogene product Raf-1 in human B-cells. Cancer Res 52(3):566, 1992

355. Taniguchi N, Kuratsune H, Kanamaru A, Tokumine Y, Tagawa S, Machii T, Kitani T: Inhibition against CFU-C and CFU-E colony formation by soluble factor(s) derived from hairy cells. Blood 73(4):907, 1989

356. Taniguchi T, Minami Y: The IL-2/IL-2 receptor system: a current overview. Cell 73:5, 1993

357. Teichmann JV, Sieber G, Ludwig WD, Ruehl H: Modulation of immune functions by long-term

treatment with recombinant interferon-alpha 2 in a patient with hairy-cell leukemia. J Interferon Res 8(1):15, 1988

358. Thaler J, Denz H, Dietze O, Gastl G, Ho AD, Gattringer C, Greil R, Lechleitner M, Huber C, Huber H: Immunohistological assessment of bone marrow biopsies from patients with hairy cell leukemia: changes following treatment with alpha-2-interferon and deoxycoformycin. Leuk Res 13(5):377, 1989

359. Thaler J, Grunewald K, Gattringer C, Ho AD, Weyrer K, Dietze O, Stauder R, Fluckinger T, Lang A, Huber H: Long-term follow-up of patients with hairy cell leukaemia treated with pentostatin: lymphocyte subpopulations and residual bone marrow infiltration. Brit J Haematol 84(1):75, 1993

360. Thiele J, Langohr J, Skorupka M, Fischer R: Reticulin fibre content of bone marrow infiltrates of malignant non-Hodgkin's lymphomas (B-cell type, low malignancy) – a morphometric evaluation before and after therapy. Virchows Arch A Pathol Anat Histopathol 417(6):485, 1990

361. Till KJ, Cawley JC: Phenotypic changes on hairy cells exposed in vitro to interferons: a quantitative FACS study. Brit J Haematol 72(3):378, 1989

362. Till KJ, Lopez A, Slupsky J, Cawley JC: C-fms protein expression by B-cells, with particular reference to the hairy cells of hairy-cell leukaemia. Brit J Haematol 83(2):223, 1993

363. Till KJ, Cawley JC: Accessory cells mediate hairy-cell proliferation by mechanism(s) involving both adhesion and TNF alpha secretion. Brit J Haematol 87(4):687, 1994

364. Till KJ, Burthem J, Lopez A, Cawley JC: Stage specific expression and function on late B cells. Blood in press

365. Tominaga T, Sho S: Alpha interferon therapy for Japanese patients with hairy cell leukaemia. Leukemia 2:554, 1988

366. Traweek ST, Sheibani K, Winberg CD, Mena RR, Wu AM, Rappaport H: Monocytoid B-cell lymphoma: its evolution and relationship to other low-grade B-cell neoplasms. Blood 73(2):573, 1989

367. Traweek ST, Sheibani K: Monocytoid B-cell lymphoma. The biologic and clinical implications of peripheral blood involvement. Am J Clin Pathol 97(4):591, 1992

368. Trentin L, Zambello R, Agostini C, Ambrosetti A, Chisesi T, Raimondi R, Bulian P, Pizzolo G, Semenzato G: Mechanisms accounting for the defective natural killer activity in patients with hairy cell leukemia. Blood 75(7):1525, 1990

369. Trentin L, Zambello R, Pizzolo G, Vinante F, Ambrosetti A, Chisesi T, Vespignani M, Feruglio C, Adami F, Agostini C, et al.: Tumor necrosis factor-alpha and B-cell growth factor induce leukemic hairy cells to proliferate in vitro. Cancer Detect Prev 15(5):385, 1991

370. Trentin L, Zambello R, Benati C, Cassatella M, Agostini C, Bulian P, Adami F, Carra G, Pizzolo G, Semenzato G: Expression and functional role of the p75 interleukin 2 receptor chain on leukemic hairy cells. Cancer Res 52(19):5223, 1992

371. Trentin L, Zambello R, Agostini C, Siviero F, Adami F, Marcolongo R, Raimondi R, Chisesi T, Pizzolo G, Semenzato G: Expression and functional role of tumor necrosis factor receptors on leukemic cells from patients with type B chronic lymphoproliferative disorders. Blood 81(3):752, 1993

372. Triozzi PL, Avery KA, Grever MR, Kraut EH: Combined effects of interferon and 2'-deoxycoformycin on 2',5'-oligoadenylate synthetase and adenosine deaminase in hairy cell and chronic lymphocytic leukemia cells. J Interferon Res 10(5):535, 1990

373. Troussard X, Flandrin G: Hairy cell leukemia. An update on a cohort of 93 patients treated in a single institution. Effects of interferon in patients relapsing after splenectomy and in patients with or without maintenance treatment. Leuk Lymphoma 14 (suppl 1):99, 1994

374. Turhan AG, Eaves CJ, Connors JM, Eaves AC, Karim KA, Silver KB: Hematologic and immunologic changes in hairy cell leukemia patients treated with alpha interferon. J Biol Regul Homeost Agents 2(4):157, 1988

375. Turner A, Kjeldsberg CR: Hairy-cell leukemia: a review. Medicine Baltimore 57:477, 1978

376. Urba WJ, Baseler MW, Kopp WC, Steis RG, Clark JW, Smith JW 2d, Coggin DL, Longo DL: Deoxycoformycin-induced immunosuppression in patients with hairy cell leukemia. Blood 73(1):38, 1989

377. VanderMolen LA, Urba WJ, Longo DL, Lawrence J, Gralnick H, Steis RG: Diffuse osteosclerosis in hairy cell leukemia. Blood 74(6):2066, 1989

378. van-Kooten C, Rensink I, Aarden L, van-Oers R: Differentiation of purified malignant B cells induced by PMA or by activated normal T cells. Leukemia 7(10):1576, 1993

379. Vardiman JW, Gilewski TA, Ratain MJ, Bitter MA, Bradlow BA, Golomb HM: Evaluation of Leu-

M5 (CD11c) in hairy cell leukemia by the alkaline phosphatase anti-alkaline phosphatase technique. Am J Clin Pathol 90(3):250, 1988

380. Vedantham S, Gamliel H, Golomb HM: Mechanism of interferon action in hairy cell leukemia: a model of effective cancer biotherapy. Cancer Res 52(5):1056, 1992

381. Visser L, Shaw A, Slupsky J, Vos H, Poppema S: Monoclonal antibodies reactive with hairy cell leukemia [see comments]. Blood 74(1):320, 1989

382. Visser L, Poppema S: Induction of B-cell chronic lymphocytic leukaemia and hairy cell leukaemia like phenotypes by phorbol ester treatment of normal peripheral blood B-cells [see comments]. Brit J Haematol 75(3):359, 1990

383. Visser L, Dabbagh L, Poppema S: Reactivity of monoclonal antibody B-ly7 with a subset of activated T cells and T-cell lymphomas. Hematol Pathol 6(1):37, 1992

384. Vonderwalde J, Mashiah A, Berrebi A: Spontaneous rupture of the spleen in hairy-cell leukemia. Clinical Oncology 7(3):241, 1981

385. von-Wussow P, Freund M, Dahle S, Jakschies D, Poliwode H, Deicher H: Immunogenicity of different types of interferons in the treatment of hairy-cell leukemia [letter]. N Engl J Med 319(18):1226, 1988

386. von-Wussow P, Pralle H, Hochkeppel HK, Jakschies D, Sonnen S, Schmidt H, Muller-Rosenau D, Franke M, Haferlach T, Zwingers T, et al.: Effective natural interferon-alpha therapy in recombinant interferon-alpha-resistant patients with hairy cell leukemia. Blood 78(1):38, 1991

387. Wagner L, Goldstone AH, Worman CP: Demonstration of the increase in serine esterase-positive T cells in hairy-cell leukemia patients undergoing alpha-interferon therapy. Leukemia 3(5):373, 1989

388. Wagner SD, Martinelli V, Luzzatto L: Similar patterns of V kappa gene usage but different degrees of somatic mutation in hairy cell leukemia, prolymphocytic leukemia, Waldenström's macroglobulinemia, and myeloma. Blood 83(12):3647, 1994

389. Ward FT, Baker J, Krishnan J, Dow N, Kjobech CH: Hairy cell leukemia in two siblings. A human leukocyte antigen-linked disease? Cancer 65(2):319, 1990

390. Watson RB, Galvani DW, Nash JR, Cawley JC: Gamma IFN receptor expression in haemic malignancies. Leuk Res 14(7):657, 1990

391. Westbrook CA, Golde DW: Autoimmune-disease in hairy-cell leukemia – clinical syndromes and treatment. Brit J Haematol 61(2):349, 1985

392. Wiernik PH, Schwartz B, Dutcher JP, Turman N, Adinolfi C: Successful treatment of hairy cell leukemia with beta-ser interferon. Am J Hematol 33(4):244, 1990

393. Wilkinson PC: The locomotor capacity of human lymphocytes and its enhancement by cell growth. Immunology 57:281, 1986

394. Wolf BC, Martin AW, Neiman RS, Janckila AJ, Yam LT, Caracansi A, Leav BA, Winpenny R, Schultz DS, Wolfe HJ: The detection of Epstein–Barr virus in hairy cell leukemia cells by in situ hybridization. Am J Pathol 136(3):717, 1990

395. Wolfe DW, Scopelliti JA, Boselli BD: Leukemic meningitis in a patient with hairy-cell leukemia – a case-report. Cancer 54(6):1085, 1984

396. Worman CP, Barker WR, Apostolov K: Saturation index of blood cell membrane fatty acids before and after IFN treatment in hairy cell leukemia. Leukemia 1:379, 1987

397. Yachnin S, Golomb HM, West EJ, Saffold C: Increased cholesterol biosynthesis in leukemic cells from patients with hairy cell leukemia. Blood 61:50, 1983

398. Yachnin S, Mannickarottu V: Increased 3-hydroxy-methylglutaryl coenzyme A reductase activity and cholesterol biosynthesis in freshly isolated hairy cell leukemia cells. Blood 63:690, 1984

399. Yam LT, Klock JC, Mielke CH: Therapeutic leukapheresis in hairy-cell leukemia – review of the literature and personal experience. Semin Oncol 11:493, 1984

400. Zafrani ES, Degos F, Guigui B, Durandschneider AM, Martin N, Flandrin G, Benhamou JP, Feldmann G: The hepatic sinusoid in hairy-cell leukemia – an ultrastructural-study of 12 cases. Human Pathology 18(8):801, 1987

401. Zauli D, Gobbi M, Crespi C, Tazzari PL, Miserocchi F, Tassinari A: Cytoskeleton organization of normal and neoplastic lymphocytes and lymphoid cell lines of T and B origin. Brit J Haematol 68(4):405, 1988

402. Zinzani PL, Lauria F, Buzzi M, Raspadori D, Gugliotta L, Bocchia M, Macchi S, Algeri R, Tura S: Hairy cell leukemia variant: a morphologic, immunologic and clinical study of 7 cases. Haematologica 75(1):54, 1990

403. Zinzani PL, Lauria F, Raspadori D, Buzzi M, Benfenati D, Bocchia M, Rondelli D, Tura S:

Comparison of low-dose versus standard-dose alpha-interferon regimen in the hairy cell leukemia treatment. Acta Haematol 85(1):16, 1991

404. Zinzani PL, Lauria F, Raspadori D, Rondelli D, Benfenati D, Pileri S, Sabattini E, Tura S: Results in hairy-cell leukemia patients treated with alpha-interferon: predictive prognostic factors. Eur J Haematol 49(3):133, 1992

405. Zola H, Siderius N, Flego L, Beckman I, Seshadri R: Cytokine receptor expression in leukaemic cells. Leuk Res 18(5):347, 1994

406. Zuzel M, Cawley JC, Paton RC, Burns GF, McNichol GP: Platelet function in hairy-cell leukaemia. J Clin Pathol 32:814, 1979

INDEX